Mariem Nouira
Hazem Ben Rayana
Samir Ennigrou

Tuberculin skin test

Mariem Nouira
Hazem Ben Rayana
Samir Ennigrou

Tuberculin skin test

Diagnostic performance for the detection of active tuberculosis

ScienciaScripts

Imprint
Any brand names and product names mentioned in this book are subject to trademark, brand or patent protection and are trademarks or registered trademarks of their respective holders. The use of brand names, product names, common names, trade names, product descriptions etc. even without a particular marking in this work is in no way to be construed to mean that such names may be regarded as unrestricted in respect of trademark and brand protection legislation and could thus be used by anyone.

Cover image: www.ingimage.com

This book is a translation from the original published under ISBN 978-620-6-72415-5.

Publisher:
Sciencia Scripts
is a trademark of
Dodo Books Indian Ocean Ltd. and OmniScriptum S.R.L publishing group

120 High Road, East Finchley, London, N2 9ED, United Kingdom
Str. Armeneasca 28/1, office 1, Chisinau MD-2012, Republic of Moldova, Europe
Printed at: see last page
ISBN: 978-620-8-32965-5

Contents

Resume

Introduction: The lymph node forms of tuberculosis often escape diagnosis by conventional tests. Our aim was to evaluate the performance of the tuberculin skin test in the diagnosis of active tuberculosis in Tunisia, using the ROC curve method.

Methodology: This was a multicentre case-control study conducted in 11 tuberculosis clinics (DATs) in Tunisia in 2014.

Results:A total of **1053** patients were included, divided into **339 cases** and **714 controls**. The mean diameter of the tuberculin TST induration was **significantly** greater in cases than in controls (13.7mm *vs.*6.2mm;$p=10^{-6}$). The area under the curve (AUC) was **0.789** [95% CI:0.758-0.819;p=0.01], which corresponds to **moderate** discriminatory power for this test. The threshold value for the diameter of the induration of the intradermal tuberculin reaction was **11 mm,** with a Youden index of 0.503. This was the most discriminating value, associated with the best sensitivity (73.7%) and specificity (76.6%).

Conclusion: We can conclude that the tuberculin skin test can be used to diagnose tuberculosis with good sensitivity and specificity. However, its interpretation and reading remain difficult and highly subjective.

I INTRODUCTION

Tuberculosis is a contagious, airborne, human-to-human infectious disease caused by a mycobacterium of the *tuberculosis* complex, which has a slow transmission cycle [1]. The main ones are *Mycobacterium tuberculosis*, also known as Koch's bacillus (BK), *Mycobacterium bovis* and *Mycobacterium africanum* [2].

Diagnosis of pulmonary tuberculosis is based on detection of the tubercle bacillus in sputum and cultures [3]. However, this method suffers from two pitfalls: firstly, this detection is often lacking in certain forms of tuberculosis (lymph node tuberculosis, meningeal tuberculosis, tuberculosis associated with HIV infection, etc.) and secondly, it does not allow tuberculosis disease to be diagnosed at an early stage, when the patient has already contaminated those around him. In this case, the diagnosis is based on a combination of epidemiological, clinical, biological and immunological factors [4].

Infection with the bacillus causes a cell-mediated immune response (delayed-type hypersensitivity) to the tuberculosis bacillus. This response can be measured and validated by the tuberculin skin test or tuberculin intradermal reaction (TIR) or Mantoux test [5].

Changes in the epidemiology of tuberculosis in Tunisia (particularly the increase in the frequency of lymph node forms at the expense of pulmonary forms) have led us to reflect on the performance of the tuberculin TST in diagnosing the disease [6, 7].

In fact, the sensitivity and specificity of the tuberculin TST are linked and vary in opposite directions (when one increases, the other decreases) [8]. This relationship could be established very clearly in the case of a test expressed by a quantitative variable, in this case the diameter of the induration of the TST.

Clearly, clinicians want a diagnostic test that is both highly sensitive and highly specific. This is not possible in practice, and a compromise must be found between sensitivity and specificity. The ROC curve (Receiver Operating Characteristic curve), originally developed to assess the informational value of radars seeking to identify an enemy attack during the Second World War, is a means of examining the relationship between the sensitivity and specificity of the tuberculin TST [9].

A practical situation frequently encountered is that of wanting to know the risk of having or not having the disease according to the result of the test. Predictive values, which depend on the prevalence of the disease in the population and express the probability of confirming the presence or absence of tuberculosis according to the results of the tuberculin TST, make it possible to estimate this risk [8].

In this study, we therefore set out to assess the performance of tuberculin TST through a multicentre case-control study.

The objectives of this work were:

- to identify discriminating thresholds for the tuberculin TST test in adult subjects aged 18 to 55, using the ROC curve method in a diagnostic situation;
- determine the likelihood ratios (positive and negative) of this test;
- to determine the positive and negative predictive values of the tuberculin TST in relation to a predefined level of tuberculosis prevalence.

II SUBJECTS AND METHODS

I.1. . Type of study

This was a multicentre, case-control, epidemiological study to evaluate the performance of tuberculin intradermo-reaction in adult subjects aged 18 to 55, during the period from 1er June 2014 to 30 November 2014.

I.2. . Study population

I.2.1. . Inclusion criteria

- Adult patients aged between 18 and 55 years with confirmed tuberculosis, recruited from 11 tuberculosis clinics (DAT) (Ariana - Tunis - Sfax - Gafsa - Ben Arous - Bizerte - Sousse - Kairouan - Sidi Bouzid - Kasserine - Tataouine), at the time of the first tuberculosis treatment in the DAT.
- Tuberculosis-free witnesses, collected in basic health centres (CSB) and/or district hospitals. All the witnesses showed no respiratory or extra-respiratory signs that could be of tuberculosis origin.

I.2.2. . Exclusion criteria

The following were excluded:

- patients already being treated for pulmonary or extra-pulmonary tuberculosis;
- patients and witnesses with a pathological condition that may lead to tuberculin anergy: acute viral infections (measles, mumps, infectious mononucleosis, influenza), lymphomas, neoplastic pathologies, sarcoidosis, severe bacterial infection, HIV infection, etc. ;
- patients and controls undergoing immunosuppressive treatment, corticosteroid therapy for more than one month or vaccination with live vaccines in the two months preceding the test;
- persons with a known history of allergic reaction to one of the components of tuberculin or to a previous administration;
- the absence of vaccine scarring in the control group.

I.2.3. . Sampling methods

The study involved intradermal tuberculin tests carried out on two separate samples:

- A sample of subjects with tuberculosis recruited consecutively in the DATs. The sample consisted of all patients consulting the aforementioned DATs during the study period, at the first remittance of their antituberculosis treatment, i.e. a total of 339 cases, divided into 158 men (46.6%) and 181 women (53.4%);
- A control sample composed of subjects free of tuberculosis consulting the CSB or the district hospital located near the DAT during the same study period. This choice was made for reasons of recruitment feasibility.

Witnesses were recruited in such a way that their sex distribution was identical to that of the tuberculosis cases. We took roughly the same proportion of males and females in the tuberculosis cases and in the witnesses. In this case, any of the male or female controls was an appropriate control for each of the male or female TB patients. The same frequency distribution according to 5-year or 10-year age groups was not possible.

We preferred this frequency matching method to the individual matching method (which consisted of choosing one or more identical witnesses for each case of tuberculosis included, in terms of the matching criteria: age, sex, place of residence) because it presented fewer practical difficulties. It would also facilitate statistical analysis. In total, we collected 714 controls, divided into 356 men (49.8%) and 358 women (50.2% of cases).

I.3. . Data collection

A data collection form with fixed items except for the location of the tuberculosis and the region, was filled in for each subject included in the study (tuberculosis patient or witness) by the same person responsible for carrying out the tuberculin DST and reading it under the supervision of a regional coordinator (appendix 1).

This form contained the following variables:

- the characteristics of the subjects: age, sex, level of education ;
- the presence of a vaccination scar (BCG);
- the absence of the exclusion criteria listed above ;
- the location of the tuberculosis;
- the date the RID was taken, the diameter of the induration (in mm), and the associated reactions: erythema, phlyctenis, necrosis or lymphangitis.

A tuberculin TST data sheet was drawn up and validated, mentioning the product used: purified tuberculin PPD (Purified Protein Derivative RT23 from Copenhagen) (appendix 2). An intradermal tuberculin reaction was performed in all subjects included in the study (tuberculosis patients and controls) by injecting 0.1 ml of tuberculin solution, strictly intradermally, into the anterior aspect of the forearm at the junction of the upper third and the lower two thirds of the forearm, at a distance from any scar.

The tuberculin TST was read after 72 hours by measuring the transverse diameter of the induration (expressed in mm) by the same member of staff at each tuberculosis clinic.

I.4. . Data capture and analysis

The data was entered and processed using SPSS version 16.0 software.

For qualitative data, we calculated simple frequencies and percentages.

To compare two percentages on two independent samples, we used Pearson's Chi-2 test.

For quantitative data, we calculated means and standard deviations when the distribution was symmetrical, quartiles (Q1: first quartile; Q3: third quartile) and a median (Q2: second quartile) when it was not. We used box plots to summarise the distribution of the diameter of the tuberculin TST induration in the patient group and in the control group [10, 11] (appendix 3).

The Student's T test was used to compare two means on two independent samples.

For all statistical tests, the significance level chosen was 0.05.

I.4.1. . Estimation of sensitivity and specificity

To assess the performance of the tuberculin TST, we first calculated the sensitivity and specificity of the TST induration diameter and the Youden index for different possible thresholds (from a TST diameter > 5 mm to a TST diameter > 15 mm).

The 95% confidence intervals ($_{CI95\%}$) for sensitivity and specificity were calculated using an Excel calculator and the properties of the exact binomial distribution [12].

Sensitivity (Se) was defined as the proportion (ranging from 0 to 1) of people with the disease who tested positive for the disease, in other words the proportion of people with the disease that the test correctly detected (true positives=TN). In contrast, the proportion of disease carriers not identified by the test were false-negative (FN) results [8, 13]:

Sensitivity

$$\text{Sensibilité} = \frac{VP}{VP + FN}$$

Specificity (Sp) was defined as the proportion (ranging from 0 to 1) of people without the disease who tested negative for the disease, in other words the proportion of people without the disease that the test determined correctly (true negatives=VN). In contrast, the proportion of disease-free subjects who tested positive were false positives (FP) [14, 15]:

Specificity

$$\text{Spécificité} = \frac{VN}{VN + FP}$$

The two intrinsic qualities of the test, sensitivity and specificity, unrelated to the population studied, have been aggregated into an index, known as the Youden index, rated J such that: J = (Se + Sp) - 1.

J varies between -1 and +1; a value of 0 or less indicates that the test is diagnostically ineffective. The better the test, the closer its Youden index is to 1 [16, 17].

The choice of the most discriminative threshold value for the induration diameter of the tuberculin TST associated with the best {sensitivity, specificity} pair was made by comparing the 95% confidence intervals (IC95%) of the sensitivity or specificity estimates for the threshold values of the tuberculin TST chosen two by two. If the 95% CIs of two sensitivity or specificity values overlapped, the two proportions were considered not significantly different and could represent the same true value in the population. On the other hand, if the respective 95% CIs did not overlap, then the statistical difference between the two proportions was considered significant.

I.4.2. . Estimation of positive and negative likelihood ratios

We calculated the positive and negative likelihood ratios of the diameter of the tuberculin TST induration for different possible thresholds (from a TST diameter > 5 mm to a TST diameter > 15 mm). Calculation of the 95% confidence intervals (95% CI) of the positive and negative likelihood ratios was also performed using the Excel calculator and the properties of the exact binomial distribution [12].

The test's likelihood ratio combines its sensitivity and specificity into a single factor [18].

The positive likelihood ratio (LR+) was defined as the ratio of the probability of a positive test result in people with the disease to the probability of the same result in people without the disease, in other words the proportion of true positives among those with the disease (i.e. sensitivity) to the proportion of false positives among those without the disease (i.e. 1 - specificity) [19, 20] :

Sensitivity

$$\text{Positive likelihood ratio} = \frac{\text{Sensibilité}}{(1 - \text{Spécificité})}$$

(1 - Specificity)

This positive likelihood ratio (LR+) varies from 0 to +TO, but in practice it varies between 1 and + TO [18]. It indicates the higher degree of probability that a person with the disease will have a positive result, compared with a person without the disease. It indicates that the better the test is able to discriminate between patients with and without the disease, the further away it is from 1 and the closer its specificity is to 1. RV+ is considered useful when its value exceeds 5 [21].

The negative likelihood ratio (LR-) was defined as the ratio of the probability of a negative test result in people with the disease to the probability of the same result in people without the disease, in other words the proportion of false negatives among people with the disease (i.e. 1 - the sensitivity) to the proportion of true negatives among people without the disease, i.e. the specificity [22] :

(1 - Sensitivity)

$$\text{Negative likelihood ratio} = \frac{(1 - \text{Sensibilité})}{\text{Spécificité}}$$

Specificity

This negative likelihood ratio (LR-), which varies between 0 and 1, indicates the greater likelihood of a person with the disease having a negative result compared with a person without the disease. The closer the LR- is to 0 and the closer the sensitivity is to 1, the better the test's ability to discriminate between those with and those without the disease. A LR- is considered useful when its value is less than 0.2 or 0.1 [23, 24].

The diagnostic contribution of a test according to the value of the positive and negative likelihood ratios is shown in Table I [21].

Table I: Diagnostic contribution of a test according to the value of the positive and negative likelihood ratios.

Positive likelihood ratio (LR+)	Negative likelihood ratio (LR-)	Diagnostic contribution
RV+ **>10**	RV- < **0.1**	**Very strong**
5 <RV+ < **10**	**0.1** < RV <0.**2**	**Fort**
2 <RV+ < **5**	**0.2<** RV <0.**5**	**Modere**
1<RV+<2	**0.5<** RV **<1**	**Low**
RV+ = **1**	RV- = **1**	**None**

I.4.3. . Estimation of the ROC curve

In order to measure the overall performance of the tuberculin TST, we used the ROC curve, from which we determined the optimal threshold value of the tuberculin TST with the best {sensitivity, specificity} ratio.

We established an ROC curve according to the diameter of the induration of the IDR, firstly by age, sex and location combined, then by age class and finally by pulmonary and lymph node location.

The ROC curve is a graphical tool used to represent the ability of a test to discriminate between the population of patients and non-diseased people.

The ROC curve represents the proportion of positive tests in the sick population (sensitivity) on the ordinate and the proportion of positive tests in the non-diseased population (specificity complement or 1 - specificity) on the abscissa, for all possible threshold values of the test. The points corresponding to the {1 - specificity, sensitivity} pairs are then placed on the graph. Their junction by straight lines leads to a trace connecting the bottom left-hand corner of the graph (sensitivity = 0 and specificity = 1) to the top right-hand corner (sensitivity = 1 and specificity = 0). This is a non-parametric construction [25 - 30].

For a test that discriminates between patients and nonpatients, it is possible to find a threshold value with 100% sensitivity and specificity. In this case, the ROC curve runs along the ordinate axis and the top of the graph.

On the other hand, if a test has zero discrimination capacity, the proportion of positives among patients will be equal to the proportion of positives among nonpatients, whatever the threshold value. In this case, the ROC curve is the diagonal line at 45°, known as the diagonal line of chance or non-information. This means that sensitivity is equal to specificity for all critical threshold values.

Most tests fall between these two extremes. A test is better the closer its ROC curve is to the top left-hand corner of the graph (Figure 1) [31, 32].

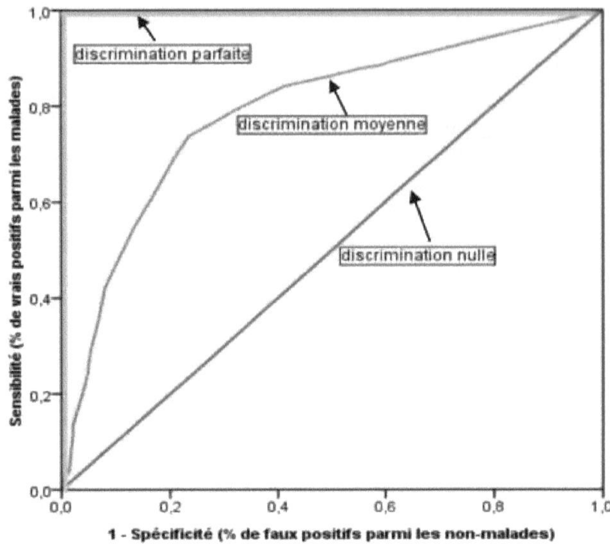

Figure 1: ROC curve or "Receiver Operating Characteristic curve", for tests with a perfect, average and zero discrimination capacity.

I.4.4. . Estimation of the area under the ROC curve

We have summarised the information contained in the ROC curve into a simple, quantitative index, the Area Under the Curve (AUC), which has the pleasant property of summarising performance for all possible discrimination thresholds [26, 33].

We calculated the AUC by age, sex and location combined, then by age group and finally by lung and lymph node location. The AUCs are presented with their 95% confidence intervals (IC95%).

The AUC is between 0.5 and 1.

When the test is perfectly discriminating, the area under the curve (AUC) is 1. This means that, given two people (one ill and the other not), the test can distinguish between the ill person and the person who is not ill in 100% of cases (Figure 2).

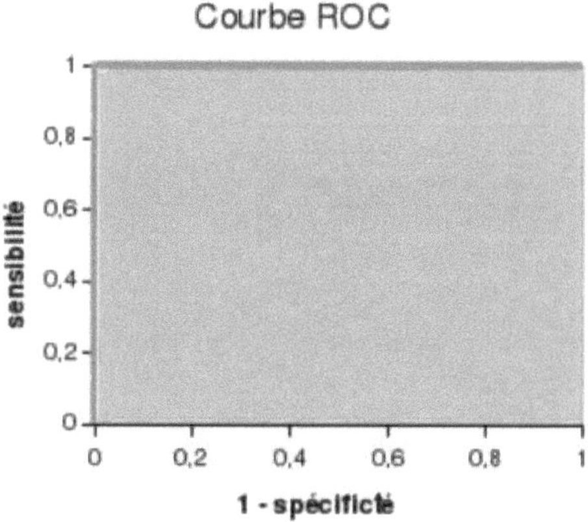

Figure 2: Area under the ROC curve for a test with perfect discriminatory power (AUC=1).

Conversely, when the test is not discriminatory, the probability of distinguishing between a sick person and a healthy person is 50% (this would be the case for a test where the result is entirely due to chance). In this case, the area under the ROC curve is 0.5 (figure 3).

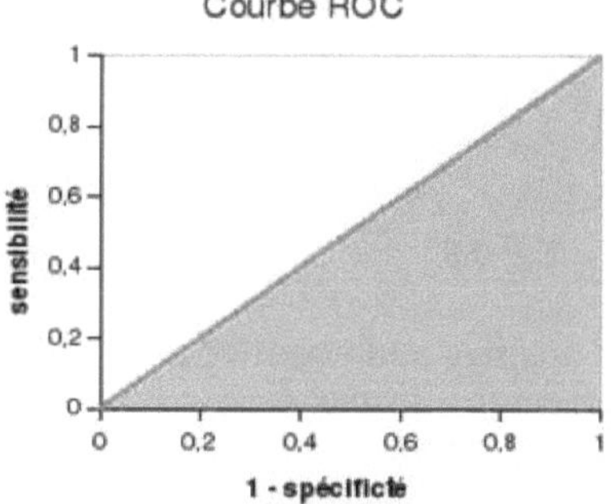

Figure 3: Area under the ROC curve for a test with no discriminatory power (AUC=0.5).

Between these two extremes, all cases are possible; the area under the curve depends on the general shape of the curve and therefore on the sensitivity and specificity of the test (figure 4). The area under the ROC curve is greater than 0.5 and close to 1, so the greater the discriminatory capacity or overall diagnostic value of a test.

An area under the ROC curve of 0.8, for example, means that a sick subject will have a better test result than a healthy subject 80% of the time.

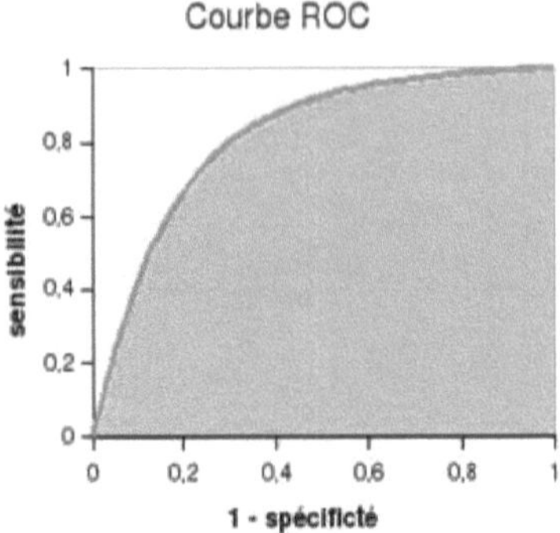

Figure 4: Area under the ROC curve for a test with good discriminatory power (0.5<AUC<1).

Using a non-parametric statistic (Mann-Withney U test), we tested the area under the ROC curve against the area under the line of non-information (null hypothesis: AUC=0.5) [9, 33]. The significance level was 0.05.

The diagnostic contribution of a test according to the value of the area under the ROC curve is shown in Table II [34].

Table II: Diagnostic contribution of a test according to the value of the area under the ROC curve.

Area under the ROC curve (AUC)	Diagnostic contribution
AUC = **1**	**Perfect**
0.9 ≤AUC< **<1**	**Fort**
0.7 ≤AUC< <0.**9**	**Modere**
0.5 ≤AUC< <0.**7**	**Low**
AUC = **0.5**	**None**

I.4.5. . Estimation of positive and negative predictive values

In order to estimate the informative contribution of the tuberculin TST, we calculated the positive predictive values (PPV) and negative predictive values (NPV) of the tuberculin TST for different possible thresholds (from a TST diameter > 5 mm to a TST diameter > 15 mm), age, sex and location combined. The 95% confidence intervals (95% CI) for the PPV and NPV were calculated using the EPITABLES program in EPI-INFO software version 6.04 (CDC/Atlanta/USA), using the properties of the exact binomial distribution.

These predictive values (also called a posteriori or post-test probabilities) were estimated firstly using the properties of Bayes' theorem [35] and secondly by establishing Fagan's nomogram [36], In both cases, it was based on the prevalence of tuberculosis (also called a priori or pre-test probability) among pneumology consultants in 3 university hospitals in Tunis (Rabta hospital in Tunis, Charles Nicolle hospital in Tunis and Abderrahmane Mami hospital in Ariana). This prevalence was estimated at around 1% in 2016.

It should be remembered that the positive predictive value (PPV) expresses the probability of being a carrier of the disease when the test is positive, and the negative predictive value (NPV) expresses the probability of being free of the disease when the test is negative, and that these latter values, with constant sensitivity (Se) and specificity (Sp), vary according to the prevalence (p) of the disease [8, 14, 37].

According to Bayes' theorem [35] :

$$VPP = \frac{Se \times p}{Se \times p + (1\text{-}Sp) \times (1\text{-}p)}$$

$$VPN = \frac{Sp \times (1\text{-}p)}{Sp \times (1\text{-}p) + (1\text{-}Se) \times p}$$

We have deduced these positive and negative predictive values (post-test probabilities) of the tuberculin TST for different possible thresholds, easily and more quickly, using a graph called Fagan's nomogram [36].

The Fagan nomogram is a graph used to estimate the positive and negative post-test probabilities (PPV and 1-VPN respectively), as a function of the pre-test probability (prevalence of the disease) in the population studied and from the positive and negative likelihood ratios. It represents respectively, on three vertical axes, with a logarithmic scale: the pre-test probability, the positive (or negative) likelihood ratio and the positive (or negative) post-test probability [38].

To apply Fagan's nomogram, we need to draw a straight line that passes through the left axis (pre-test probability), the central axis (positive or negative likelihood ratio) and then crosses the right axis to determine the post-test probability (blue line for RV+ and VPP and red line for RV- and 1-VPN).

An example of the use of this nomogram is shown in Figure 5 [39].

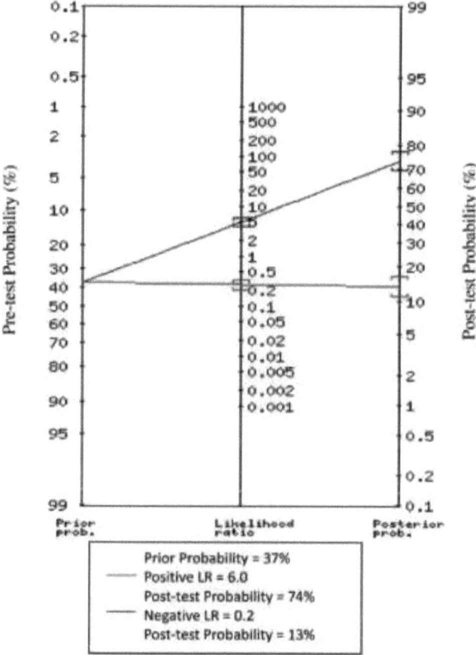

Figure 5: Example of the Fagan nomogram.

I.5. . Bibliographic research :

The bibliographic search was carried out using PubMed, Sciences Direct and the Google Scholar search engine with the following key words: tuberculosis, tuberculin test, case-control studies, ROC curve.

I.6. . Ethical considerations :

In this study to evaluate the performance of the tuberculin TST, particularly in controls, verbal agreement was obtained after explaining the purpose of the study. They were informed of their right to refuse and of the strict confidentiality of the information collected.

III RESULTS

I.7. 1. Descriptive characteristics of patients and witnesses

I.7.1. 1. According to age

The mean age of the patients was 38.3 years (standard deviation: 11.8) with extremes ranging from 18 to 55 years. The mean age of the controls was 33.6 years (standard deviation: 11) with extremes ranging from 18 to 55 years.

Figure 6 shows the age distribution of patients and controls respectively.

In the control group, the typical age group was 20-29 years (41.8%). Among patients, the least represented age group was under 20 (5.7%).

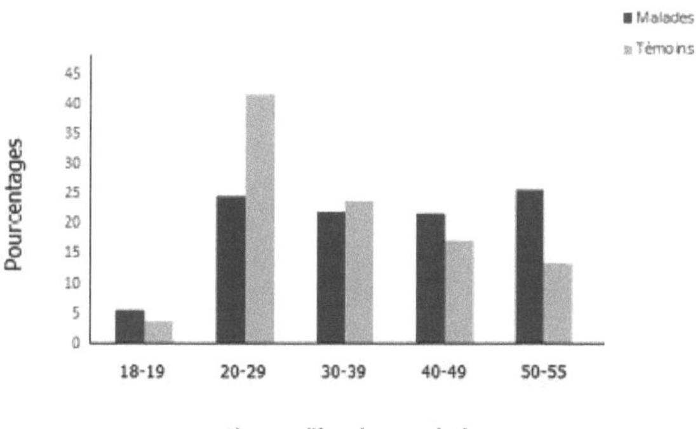

Figure n°6 : Distribution of patients (n=336) and controls (n=706) by age group.

I.7.2. 2. By gender

In the group of tuberculosis patients, 46.6% of subjects were male, giving a male/female sex ratio of 0.87. In the control group, 50.2% of subjects were female, giving a sex ratio of 0.99:1.

I.7.3. 3. Depending on whether or not there is a BCG scar

The BCG scar was present in 83.8% of tuberculosis patients. It was present in all controls.

I.7.4. 4. By level of education

Illiteracy was significantly higher in the patient group than in the control group (16.8% versus 4.1%; $p=10^{-6}$). For the higher level, controls were significantly more represented (32.8% versus 14.1%; $p=10^{-6}$) (Figure 7).

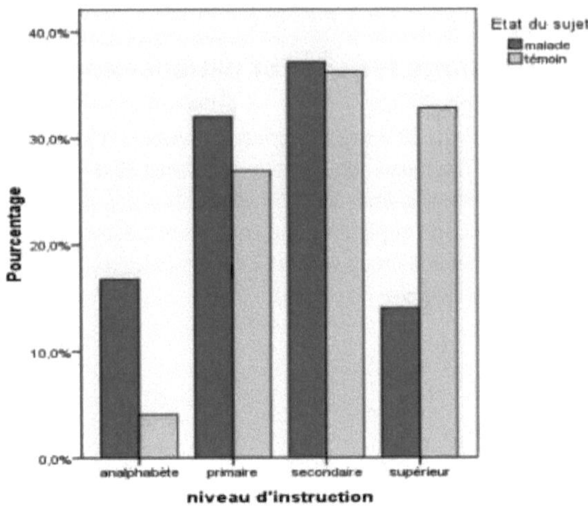

Figure 7: Distribution of patients (n=334) and controls (n=713) by level of education.

I.7.5. 5. By geographical location

Figures 8 and 9 show the distribution of patients and witnesses by geographical location. The regions of Ben Arous and Tataouine were the least represented: 2.5% and 3.5% respectively in the group of patients and 4.3% and 5% respectively in the group of witnesses.

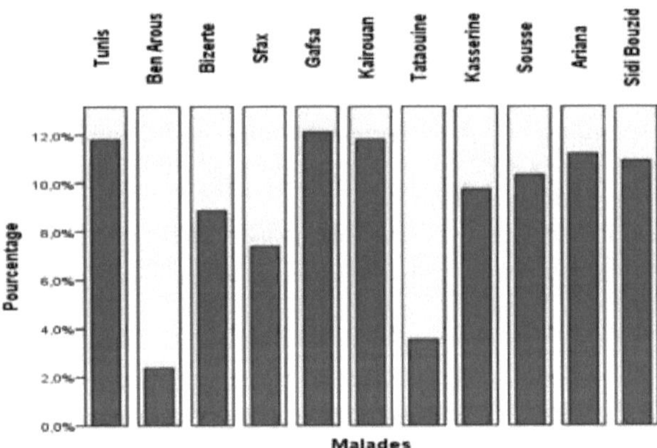

Figure 8: Distribution of patients (n=339) by geographical location.

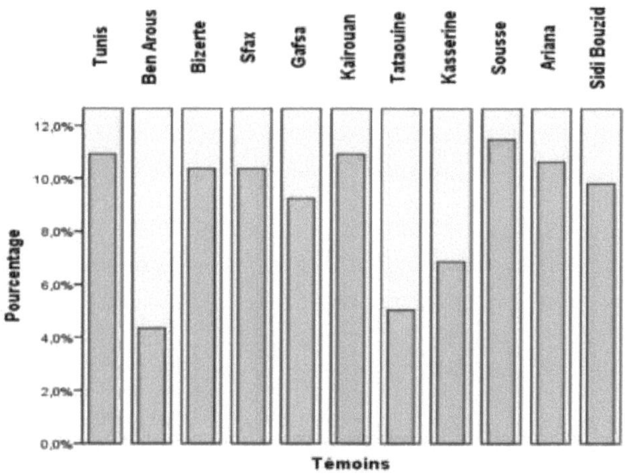

Figure 9: Breakdown of respondents (n=714) by geographical location.

I.8. 2. Characteristics of patients according to the location of the tuberculosis

Lymph nodes accounted for 53.3% of all tuberculosis patients, followed by the lungs (35.7%) and the pleura (5.6%) (Figure 10).

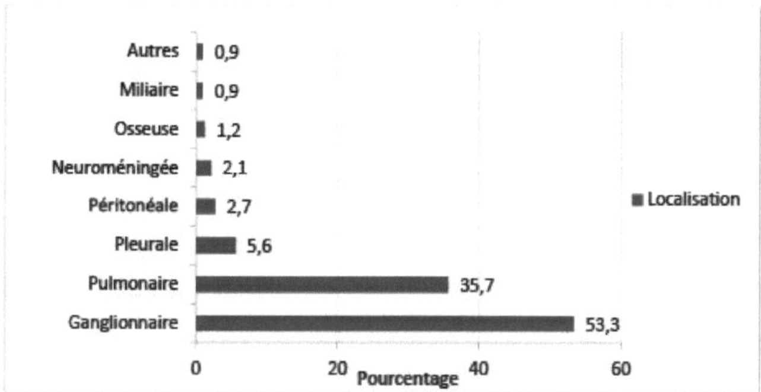

Figure 10: Distribution of patients (n=339) according to the location of the tuberculosis.

I.9. 3. Results of the tuberculin test

I.9.1. 1 Positional parameters and dispersion of the IDR diameter in the two groups

In patients, the mean diameter of the tuberculin DST induration was 13.7 mm (standard deviation: 0.7) with extremes ranging from 0 to 30 mm. In controls, the mean diameter of the tuberculin DST induration was 6.2 mm (standard deviation: 6.4) with extremes ranging from 0 to 28 mm. The difference was statistically significant (p=10).$^{-6}$

Figure 11 shows the distribution of patients and controls respectively according to the diameter

of the induration of the tuberculin TST.
In the patient group, the two modal classes of induration diameter were 10-14 mm and 15-19 mm (28.6% and 28.6% respectively). In the control group, it was 0-4 mm (45.2%).

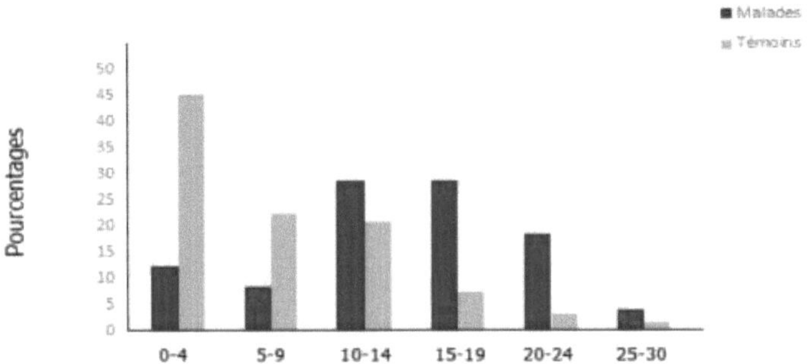

Figure 11: Distribution of patients (n=339) and controls (n=714) according to the diameter of the induration on the tuberculin DST.

The median diameter of the induration on the tuberculin TST was 15 mm in patients and 5 mm in controls (Figure 12).

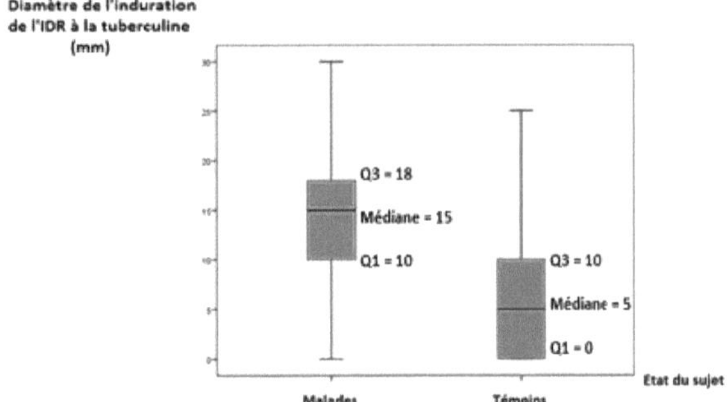

Figure 12: Box plot of the distribution of patients (n=339) and controls (n=714) according to the diameter of the induration of the TST.

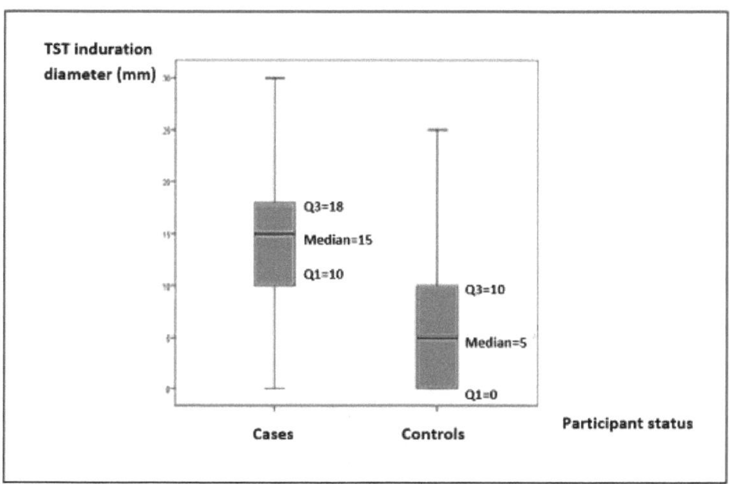

Figure 1. Box plot of TST diameter for cases and controls

I.9.2. 2. Results of the ROC curve

I.9.2.1. 1. According to the diameter of the IDR induration, age, sex and location combined

The overall performance of the tuberculin TST according to the diameter of the induration was measured by the ROC curve (Figure 13).

The Area Under the Curve (AUC) was 0.789 [95% CI: 0.758 - 0.819; p=0.01].

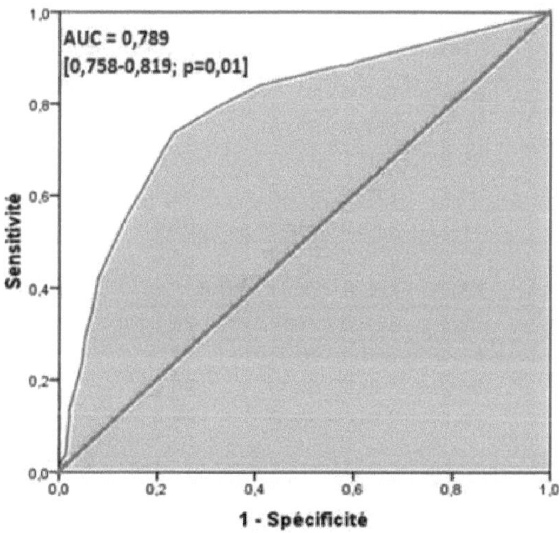

Figure 13: ROC curve measuring the performance of tuberculin TST according to the diameter of the induration, age, sex and location combined.

I.9.2.1.1. 1. Values of sensitivity (Se), specificity (Sp) and De Youden index corresponding to different possible thresholds

When comparing TST cut-off values of 5, 6 and 7 mm, there was no significant gain in sensitivity (the confidence intervals overlapped).

When comparing the TST cut-off value of greater than or equal to 7 mm with the cut-off value of greater than or equal to 10 mm, there was no significant gain in sensitivity either (the confidence intervals overlapped).
A cut-off value greater than or equal to 10 mm [95% CI for specificity: 64.1% - 70.9%] was significantly less specific than a cut-off value greater than or equal to 11 mm [95% CI for specificity: 73.3% - 79.5%] (confidence intervals did not overlap), but not significantly more sensitive.
When comparing the threshold value of the TST greater than or equal to 11 mm with the threshold value greater than or equal to 12 mm, there was no significant gain in sensitivity: [95% CI: 68.8% - 78.1%] versus [95% CI: 64.2% - 73.9%] (the confidence intervals overlapped) and no gain in specificity: [95% CI: 73.3% - 79.5%] versus [95% CI: 76% - 81.9%] (the confidence intervals overlapped).
The cut-off value for RDI diameter greater than or equal to 10 mm was worse than the cut-off value greater than or equal to 11 mm.
The cut-off value for the diameter of the induration in the TST, which was the most discriminatory, associated with the best sensitivity (73.7%) and specificity (76.6%) ratio, was therefore 11 mm with a Youden index of 0.503 (table III).

I.9.2.1.2. 2. Likelihood ratio (LR) values corresponding to different possible thresholds

For the threshold value of TST diameter greater than or equal to 11 mm, the positive likelihood ratio was 3.1 [95% CI: 2.7 - 3.6] and the negative likelihood ratio was 0.34 [95% CI: 0.28 - 0.41] (table IV).

Table III: Sensitivity, specificity and Youden index of the induration diameter of the tuberculin TST for different possible thresholds.

Diameter of IDR induration >= a (mm)	Sensitivity (%)	95% CI	Specificity (%)	95% CI	Youden index (J)
5	87,6	[83,6 - 90,7]	45,2	[41,4 - 48,7]	0,328
6	86,1	[82,0 - 89,4]	50,8	[47,1 - 54,4]	0,369
7	85,0	[80,7 - 83,3]	55,6	[51,9 - 59,2]	0,406
8	84,1	[79,8 - 87,5]	58,9	[55,3 - 62,5]	0,430
9	81,1	[76,6 - 84,9]	64,4	[60,8 - 67,8]	0,455
10	79,4	[74,7 - 83,3]	67,6	[64,1 - 70,9]	0,470
11	**73,7**	[68,8 - 78,1]	**76,6**	[73,3 - 79,5]	**0,503**
12	69,3	[64,2 - 73,9]	79,1	[76,0 - 81,9]	0,484
13	61,4	[56,0 - 66,4]	83,1	[80,1 - 85,6]	0,445
14	54,9	[49,5 - 60,1]	86,6	[83,9 - 88,9]	0,415
15	50,7	[45,4 - 56,0]	88,4	[85,8 - 90,5]	0,391

CI: confidence interval

Table IV: Likelihood ratios of the diameter of the induration of the tuberculin for different possible thresholds.

Diameter of IDR induration >= a (mm)	Positive likelihood ratio (LR+)	95% CI	Negative likelihood ratio (LR-)	95% CI
5	1,6	[1,5 - 1,7]	0,27	[0,20 - 0,37]
6	1,7	[1,6 - 1,9]	0,27	[0,21 - 0,36]
7	1,9	[1,7 - 2,1]	0,27	[0,20 - 0,35]

8	2,0	[1,9 - 2,3]	0,27	[0,21 - 0,34]
9	2,3	[2,0 - 2,6]	0,29	[0,23 - 0,37]
10	2,4	[2,2 - 2,8]	0,30	[0,25 - 0,38]
11	**3,1**	[2,7 - 3,6]	**0,34**	[0,28 - 0,41]
12	3,3	[2,8 - 3,9]	0,39	[0,33 - 0,46]
13	3,6	[3,0 - 4,3]	0,46	[0,40 - 0,53]
14	4,1	[3,3 - 5,0]	0,52	[0,46 - 0,59]
15	4,4	[3,5 - 5,5]	0,56	[0,50 - 0,62]

I.9.2.2. 2. According to the diameter of the induration of the IDR and the age class

We chose to divide the subjects into two age groups: those aged under 35 and those aged 35 and over (the mean age of all subjects). For subjects aged under 35 (148 patients and 441 controls), the threshold value for the diameter of the induration of the TST, associating the best combination of sensitivity (79.1%) and specificity (79.8%) was 11 mm with a Youden index of 0.589. For subjects aged 35 and over (188 patients and 265 controls), the threshold value for the diameter of the induration of the TST, associating the best sensitivity (70.2%) and specificity (71.3%), was 11 mm with a Youden index of 0.415. Tables V and VI summarise the results of the ROC curve according to age group.

Table V: Values of sensitivity, specificity, Youden index and positive and negative likelihood ratios corresponding to different possible thresholds for subjects aged under 35.

Diameter of IDR induration >= a (mm)	Sensitivity (%) 95% CI	Specificity (%) 95% CI	Youden index (J)	RV+ 95% CI	RV- 95% CI
5	91,2 [85,5 - 94,7]	49,2 [44,5 - 53,8]	0,404	1,8 [1,6 - 2,0]	0,18 [0,10 - 0,30]
6	89,9 [83,9 - 93,7]	54,6 [49,9 - 59,2]	0,445	2,0 [1,8 - 2,3]	0,19 [0,11 - 0,30]
7	87,8 [81,5 - 92,1]	59,1 [54,5 - 63,6]	0,469	2,1 [1,9 - 2,4]	0,20 [0,13 - 0,32]
8	87,2 [80,8 - 91,6]	62,3 [57,7 - 66,7]	0,495	2,3 [2,0 - 2,6]	0,20 [0,13 - 0,31]
9	84,5 [77,7 - 89,4]	67,1 [62,6 - 71,3]	0,516	2,6 [2,2 - 3,0]	0,23 [0,16 - 0,34]
10	81,8 [74,7 - 87,1]	70,5 [66,1 - 74,5]	0,523	2,8 [2,4 - 3,3]	0,26 [0,18 - 0,37]
11	**79,1** [71,8 - 84,8]	**79,8** [75,8 - 83,3]	**0,589**	**3,9** [3,2 - 4,8]	**0,26** [0,19 - 0,36]
12	71,6 [63,8 - 78,2]	82,0 [78,2 - 85,3]	0,536	4,0 [3,2 - 5,0]	0,35 [0,27 - 0,45]
13	62,2 [54,1 - 69,6]	83,9 [80,2 - 87,0]	0,461	3,9 [3,0 - 4,9]	0,45 [0,36 - 0,56]
14	55,4 [47,4 - 63,2]	88,0 [84,6 - 90,7]	0,434	4,6 [3,4 - 6,2]	0,51 [0,42 - 0,61]
15	51,4 [43,4 - 59,3]	89,6 [86,4 - 92,1]	0,410	4,9 [3,6 - 6,7]	0,54 [0,46 - 0,64]
Area under the curve (AUC): 0.822; **95% CI:** 0 p (significance level) = 0.02.			,782 - 0,862.		

Table VI: Values of sensitivity, specificity, Youden index and positive and

negative likelihood ratios corresponding to different possible thresholds for subjects aged 35 and over.

Diameter of IDR induration >= a (mm)	Sensitivity (%) 95% CI	Specificity (%) 95% CI	Youden index (J)	RV+ 95% CI	RV- 95% CI
5	85,1 [79,3 - 89,4]	38,1 [32,4 - 44,0]	0,232	1,4 [1,2 - 1,5]	0,39 [0,27 - 0,57]
6	83,5 [77,5 - 88,1]	44,2 [38,3 - 50,1]	0,277	1,5 [1,3 - 1,7]	0,37 [0,26 - 0,53]
7	83,0 [76,9 - 87,6]	49,0 [43,0 - 55,0]	0,320	1,6 [1,4 - 1,9]	0,35 [0,25 - 0,49]
8	81,9 [75,7 - 86,7]	52,8 [46,8 - 58,7]	0,347	1,7 [1,5 - 2,0]	0,34 [0,25 - 0,47]
9	78,7 [72,3 - 83,9]	59,6 [53,6 - 65,3]	0,383	1,9 [1,7 - 2,3]	0,36 [0,27 - 0,48]
10	77,7 [71,1 - 83,0]	62,6 [56,6 - 68,2]	0,403	2,1 [1,7 - 2,5]	0,36 [0,27 - 0,47]
11	**70,2** [63,3 - 76,2]	**71,3** [65,6 - 76,4]	**0,415**	**2,4** [2,0 - 3,0]	**0,41** [0,33 - 0,53]
12	68,1 [61,1 - 74,3]	74,3 [68,7 - 79,2]	0,424	2,6 [2,1 - 3,3]	0,43 [0,34 - 0,53]
13	61,2 [54,0 - 67,8]	81,5 [76,4 - 85,7]	0,427	3,3 [2,5 - 4,4]	0,47 [0,39 - 0,57]
14	54,8 [47,6 - 61,7]	83,8 [78,9 - 87,7]	0,386	3,4 [2,5 - 4,6]	0,54 [0,46 - 0,64]
15	51,1 [43,4 - 58,1]	86,0 [81,3 - 89,7]	0,371	3,7 [2,6 - 5,1]	0,57 [0,49 - 0,66]
Area under the curve (AUC): 0.750**; 95% CI:** p = 0.02.			0,703 - 0,798.		

I.9.2.3. 3. Depending on the diameter of the induration of the IDR and the location

We measured the performance of tuberculin TST for pulmonary and lymph node localisation. For the pulmonary site (121 patients and 714 controls), the threshold value for the diameter of the induration of the TST, with the best combination of sensitivity (70.2%) and specificity (76.6%), was 11 mm with a Youden index of 0.468.

For lymph node localisation (180 patients and 714 controls), the threshold value for the diameter of the induration of the TST, with the best combination of sensitivity (77.8%) and specificity (76.6%), was also 11 mm, with a Youden index of 0.544.

Figures 14 and 15 and tables VII and VIII show the results of the ROC curve as follows the location of the tuberculosis.

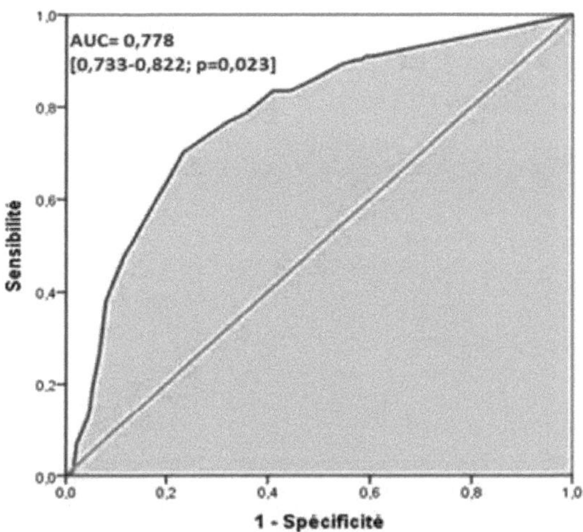

Figure 14: ROC curve measuring the performance of the tuberculin TST according to the diameter of the induration and the location in the lung.

Table VII: Values for sensitivity, specificity, Youden index and positive and negative likelihood ratios corresponding to different possible thresholds for pulmonary localisation.

Diameter of IDR induration >= a (mm)	Sensitivity (%) 95% CI	Specificity (%) 95% CI	Youden index (J)	RV+ 95% CI	RV- 95% CI
5	89,3 [82,4 - 93,6]	45,2 [41,6 - 48,9]	0,345	1,6 [1,5 - 1,8]	0,22 [0,13 - 0,38]
6	86,0 [78,6 - 91,0]	50,8 [47,1 - 54,4]	0,368	1,7 [1,6 - 1,9]	0,28 [0,18 - 0,43]
7	83,5 [75,8 - 89,0]	55,6 [51,9 - 59,2]	0,391	1,9 [1,7 - 2,1]	0,30 [0,20 - 0,45]
8	83,5 [75,8 - 89,0]	58,9 [55,3 - 62,5]	0,424	2,0 [1,8 - 2,3]	0,28 [0,19 - 0,42]
9	78,5 [70,3 - 84,8]	64,4 [60,8 - 67,8]	0,429	2,2 [1,9 - 2,5]	0,33 [0,24 - 0,47]
10	76,9 [68,5 - 83,4]	67,6 [64,1 - 70,9]	0,445	2,4 [2,0 - 2,8]	0,34 [0,25 - 0,48]
11	**70,2** [61,5 - 77,6]	**76,6** [73,3 - 79,5]	**0,468**	**3,0** [2,5 - 3,6]	**0,39** [0,29 - 0,51]
12	65,3 [56,4 - 73,1]	79,1 [76,0 - 81,9]	0,444	3,1 [2,6 - 3,8]	0,44 [0,34 - 0,56]
13	57,9 [48,9 - 66,3]	83,1 [80,1 - 85,6]	0,410	3,4 [2,7 - 4,3]	0,51 [0,41 - 0,63]
14	51,2 [42,4 - 60,0]	86,6 [83,9 - 88,9]	0,378	3,8 [2,9 - 4,9]	0,56 [0,47 - 0,68]
15	47,9 [39,2 -	88,4 [85,8 -	0,363	4,1 [3,1 -	0,59 [0,50 -

	56,8]	90,5]		5,4]	0,70]

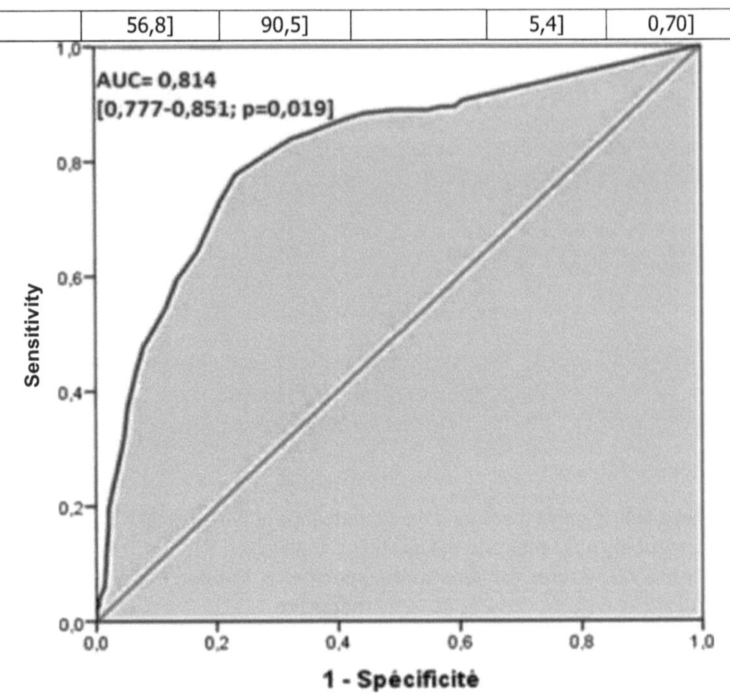

Figure 15: ROC curve measuring the performance of the tuberculin TST according to the diameter of the induration and the lymph node location.

Table VIII: Values for sensitivity, specificity, Youden index and positive and negative likelihood ratios corresponding to different possible thresholds for lymph node localisation.

Diameter of IDR induration >= a (mm)	Sensitivity (%) 95% CI	Specificity (%) 95% CI	Youden index (J)	RV+ 95% CI	RV- 95% CI
5	88,9 [83,4 - 92,6]	45,2 [41,4 - 48,7]	0,341	1,6 [1,5 - 1,8]	0,25 [0,16 - 0,37]
6	88,9 [83,4 - 92,6]	50,8 [47,0 - 54,3]	0,397	1,8 [1,6 - 2,0]	0,22 [0,14 - 0,33]
7	88,3 [82,8 - 92,2]	55,6 [51,9 - 59,2]	0,439	2,0 [1,8 - 2,2]	0,21 [0,14 - 0,32]
8	87,2 [81,5 - 91,3]	58,9 [55,3 - 62,5]	0,461	2,1 [1,9 - 2,4]	0,22 [0,15 - 0,32]
9	85,0 [79,0 - 89,4]	64,4 [60,8 - 67,8]	0,494	2,4 [2,1 - 2,7]	0,23 [0,16 - 0,33]
10	83,9 [77,8 - 88,5]	67,6 [64,1 - 70,9]	0,515	2,6 [2,3 - 2,9]	0,24 [0,17 - 0,33]
11	**77,8**	**76,6**	**0,544**	**3,3**	**0,29**

	[71,1 - 83,2]	[73,3 - 79,5]		[2,8 - 3,9]	[0,22 - 0,38]
12	73,3 [66,4 - 79,2]	79,1 [76,0 - 81,9]	0,524	3,5 [3,0 - 4,2]	0,34 [0,26 - 0,43]
13	64,4 [57,2 - 71,1]	83,1 [80,1 - 85,6]	0,475	3,8 [3,1 - 4,6]	0,43 [0,35 - 0,52]
14	59,4 [52,1 - 66,3]	86,6 [83,9 - 88,9]	0,460	4,4 [3,5 - 5,5]	0,47 [0,39 - 0,56]
15	54,4 [47,1 - 61,5]	88,4 [85,8 - 90,5]	0,428	4,7 [3,7 - 6,0]	0,51 [0,44 - 0,60]

I.9.3. 3. Estimation of the predictive values of the tuberculin TST corresponding to different possible thresholds on the basis of the prevalence among pneumology consultants in three hospitals in the greater Tunis area.

Table IX summarises the results of the positive and negative predictive values calculated using Bayes' theorem and the Fagan nomogram. For the upper threshold value
or equal to 11 mm (age, sex and location combined), the positive predictive value (PPV) and negative predictive value (NPV) calculated using Bayes' theorem were 3.11% and 99.52% respectively, and those calculated using Fagan's nomogram were 3.11% and 99.52% respectively (figure 16). The Fagan nomograms for the other possible thresholds for the IDR induration diameter are shown in Figures 17 to 26 in Appendix 4.

Table IX: Positive predictive values (PPV) **and negative predictive values** (NPV) **calculated**
using Bayes' theorem and the Fagan nomogram corresponding to different possible thresholds

Diameter of IDR induration >= a (mm)	PPV (%) 95% CI (Bayes Theorem)	VPN (%) 95% CI (Bayes Theorem)	PPV (%) 95% CI (Fagan Nomogram)	NPV (%) 95% CI (Fagan Nomogram)
5	1,59 [0,80 - 2,84]	99,72 [98,48 - 100,00]	1,70 [0,9 - 3,02]	99,72 [98,48 - 100,00]
6	1,71 [0,85 - 3,04]	99,75 [98,64 - 100,00]	1,86 [0,96 - 3,23]	99,75 [98,64 - 100,00]
7	1,81 [0,91 - 3,22]	99,77 [98,76 - 100,00]	1,81 [0,91 - 3,22]	99,77 [98,76 - 100,00]
8	2,07 [1,07 - 3,59]	99,36 [98,16 - 99,86]	2,02 [1,07 - 3,59]	99,78 [98,83 - 100,00]
9	2,26 [1,17 - 3,92]	99,61 [98,62 - 99,95]	2,07 [1,04 - 3,69]	99,61 [98,62 - 99,95]
10	2,40 [1,24 - 4,15]	99,63 [98,69 - 99,95]	2,00 [0,96 - 3,64]	99,63 [98,69 - 99,95]
11	**3,11** [1,67 - 5,27]	**99,52** [98,62 - 99,90]	**3,11** [1,67 - 5,27]	**99,52** [98,62 - 99,90]
12	3,12 [1,62 - 5,39]	99,55 [98,69 - 99,90]	3,38 [1,81 - 5,71]	99,55 [98,69 - 99,90]
13	3,64 [1,89 - 6,28]	99,44 [98,59 - 99,84]	3,64 [1,89 - 6,28]	99,44 [98,59 - 99,84]

14	3,90 [1,96 - 6,87]	99,35 [98,49 - 99,78]	4,25 [2,21 - 7,31]	99,48 [98,67 - 99,85]
15	4,31 [2,17 - 7,58]	99,37 [98,54 - 99,79]	4,31 [2,17 - 7,58]	99,37 [98,54 - 99,79]

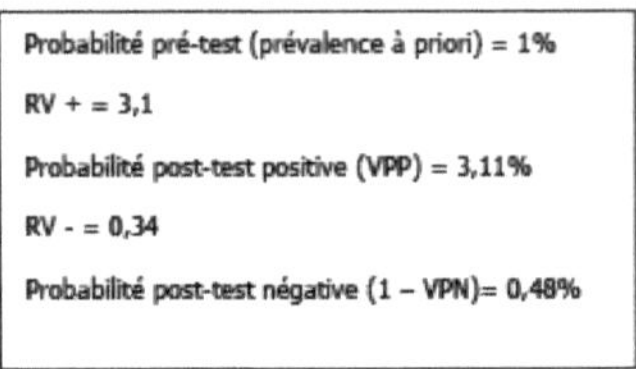

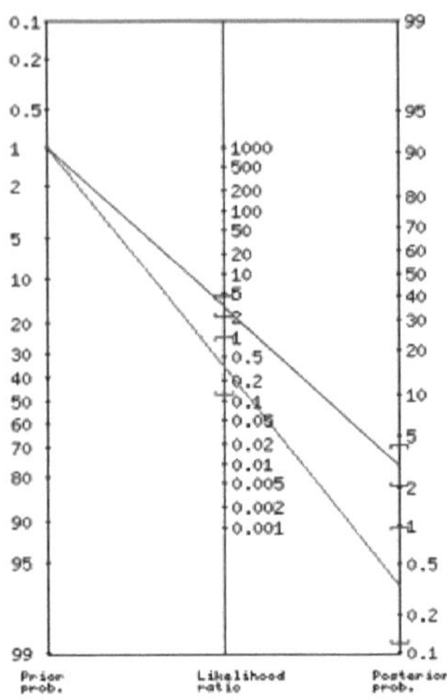

Probability pre-test (prevalence a priori) = 1%
RV + = 3.1
Probability post-test positive (PPV) = 3.11%.
RV - = 0.34
Probability post-test negative (1 - VPN)= 0,48%

Figure 16: Positive predictive value (PPV) and negative predictive value (NPV) based on the Fagan

Fagan nomogram for the threshold value of TST induration greater than or equal to 11 mm, age, sex and location combined.

I.9.4. 4. Summary of results

- The threshold of 11 mm for the diameter of the induration on the tuberculin TST was the discriminating threshold, irrespective of age, sex and location.
- For the threshold value of the diameter of the TST greater than or equal to 11 mm, the positive likelihood ratio was equal to 3.1; the negative likelihood ratio was equal to 0.34; the area under the ROC curve was 0.789, which corresponds to moderate discriminatory power for this test.
- The predictive values calculated using Bayes' theorem and established on the basis of Fagan's nomogram were comparable and valid only for subjects consulting a lung specialist.

IV DISCUSSION

The tuberculin test or TST is useful both for diagnosing and screening for tuberculosis infection, and for studying the delayed hypersensitivity reaction induced by BCG vaccination [40].

It is a measurable and valid test, and its threshold of positivity is a criterion for judging whether the test is negative or positive. However, mere knowledge of the sensitivity and specificity of the TST obtained for a single particular threshold of use is insufficient to describe the discriminatory power of this instrument, which is defined by its ability to differentiate between diseased and non-diseased subjects in comparison with the gold standard or reference test [24]. Tuberculin TST results are quantitative. In this case, the result is formulated in the form of a numerical value, which is the result of reading the diameter of the induration of the TST. It is therefore necessary to set a threshold at which this result is considered positive. Determining this threshold is not easy. If it is too low, many healthy people will be considered to be ill, leading to many false positives. On the other hand, if the threshold is too high, many sick people will be considered healthy, leading to many false negatives. Thus, for each fixed threshold, a quantitative test will have different sensitivity and specificity [24, 28, 29].

To determine the optimum threshold with the best {sensitivity, specificity} combination, the so-called ROC curve (Receiver Operating Characteristic) is used. This curve is a graphical representation of the relationship between sensitivity and specificity [31].

The information contained in the ROC curve can be summarised in a simple, quantitative index: the Area Under the Curve (AUC), which has the pleasant property of summarising performance for all possible discrimination thresholds.

The two characteristics, sensitivity and specificity, are intrinsic to the test and do not relate to the population. They therefore do not provide an answer to an important question for the doctor and the patient: what is the probability of being ill in the presence of a positive test? (or what is the probability of not being ill in the presence of a negative test?) [37].

Likelihood ratios and positive and negative predictive values are better indices in this case for assessing the diagnostic contribution of a positive or negative tuberculin TST result. These predictive values depend closely on the frequency of the disease (or prevalence) in the population studied [24].

In this study, we therefore set out to assess the performance of tuberculin TST through a multicentre case-control study during the period from 1er June 2014 to 30 November 2014.

The objectives of this work were:

- to identify discriminating thresholds for tuberculin TST in adults aged 18 to 55, using the ROC curve method in diagnostic situations,
- determine the likelihood ratios (positive and negative) of this test,
- determine positive and negative predictive values based on a predefined prevalence level.

IV.1. Sampling methods

In our study, we worked on two separate samples: a group of 339 patients with tuberculosis and a group of 714 controls without tuberculosis.

Patients with confirmed tuberculosis were recruited from 11 anti-tuberculosis clinics (Ariana - Tunis - Sfax - Gafsa - Ben Arous - Bizerte - Sousse - Kairouan - Sidi Bouzid - Kasserine - Tataouine), at the time of the first delivery of anti-tuberculosis treatment in the DAT. The tuberculosis-free witnesses, with the same gender distribution, were collected from basic health centres and/or district hospitals.

In both groups, the subjects recruited were aged between 18 and 55. The choice of this age range reduces the risk of misinterpretation of the tuberculin TST. These would be caused by

prior BCG vaccination less than 5 years old (for children) and immune deficiency (for elderly subjects) [41].
Excluding children and subjects aged over 55 from our study reduces the number of false positives and false negatives.
In a study carried out by Lee et al in South Korea [42], the aim was to compare two commercially available Quantiferon tests: QuantiFERON TB-Gold® and T-SPOT.TB® (Quantiferon tests are an alternative to the tuberculin TST for the diagnosis of latent tuberculosis infection, by detecting the release of interferon γ [43]), 218 subjects were recruited from a university hospital in South Korea between July 2004 and June 2005. They were divided into two groups: 87 with active tuberculosis and 131 with a low risk of developing tuberculosis (healthy subjects, correctly vaccinated subjects, students with normal X-rays and no history of tuberculosis). The sampling methods used were consistent with those used in our study (case-control study). However, the sample selected was smaller than in our study (218 subjects for the two groups versus 1053 subjects in our study). Subjects ranged in age from 15 to 80 years, despite a vaccination profile similar to that in our country.
In the Moroccan study carried out by Nayme et al [44], the aim of which was to determine a threshold of positivity of the tuberculin DST above which the probability of tuberculosis infection or disease is high, tuberculin tests were carried out in 174 patients with confirmed tuberculosis and 205 control subjects collected at the Moulay Youssef hospital of the "Ibn Sina" university hospital centre in Rabat. The sampling methods were consistent with those used in our study, particularly in the choice of case and control groups. However, the size of the sample selected was smaller than in our study (379 subjects for the two groups versus 1053 subjects in our study).
In a Japanese study conducted by Mori et al [45], the aim was to demonstrate the value of a Quantiferon test using the CFP-10 (Complement Factor P) and ESAT-6 (Early Secretory Antigenic Target produced by *myobacterium tuberculosis*) antigens in the diagnosis of tuberculosis in vaccinated subjects, The study sample consisted of 216 trainee nurses with no identified risk of tuberculosis recruited from different universities and 152 subjects suspected of having tuberculosis who had received anti-tuberculosis treatment for less than a week recruited from different hospitals. This was a case-control study similar to our study conducted over 4 months from July to October 2002. However, the sample size was small compared with our study (368 subjects for both groups versus 1053 subjects in our study).
In Spain, Altet et al [46] selected a sample of 1335 subjects who were close contacts of 103 tuberculosis patients declared between 2007 and 2009 and who had been exposed to tuberculosis for at least 6 hours per week in a prospective 4-year study designed to compare the value of QuantiFERON TB-Gold® and the tuberculin TST in predicting tuberculosis disease. These subjects had undergone a tuberculin test during their first visit, and were then followed up for 4 years and immediately treated if tuberculosis was suspected during this period.
Diel et al [47] conducted a 2-year prospective study in Germany. The aim of the study was to compare the results of QuantiFERON TB-Gold® and tuberculin TST in the diagnosis of tuberculosis. The study sample consisted of 601 close contacts of subjects with declared tuberculosis between May 2005 and April 2006. These subjects had undergone tuberculin testing for the first 8 weeks, after which the course of the disease was monitored for 2 years.
This sampling method, based on prospective data collection, appears to be more effective than ours, allowing better control of bias and risk factors through continuous monitoring of subjects. However, this prospective approach depends on the country's infrastructure, its degree of development and the level of education of the subjects studied, which would make it difficult

to use such a large sample in our country.

In the Danish study conducted by Brock et al [48], the aim of which was to compare the performance of the tuberculin TST and the QuantiFERON TB-Gold® in detecting latent tuberculosis, the sample consisted of 125 Danish students who were contacts of a declared tuberculosis patient. The students were divided into two groups according to the degree of exposure to the ill subject: 85 subjects recruited were close contacts of the index subject (classmates in the same class or contacts living with him in the same household) and 40 subjects recruited were students from two other classes in the same school who were not close to the index subject. In this study, the influence of vaccination on the interpretation of the tuberculin TST was taken into account (all the subjects recruited were unvaccinated).

IV.2 Descriptive characteristics of the subjects surveyed

IV.2.1. Characteristics according to age, sex ratio and presence or absence of BCG scarring

The mean age of the patients was 38.3 years (standard deviation: 11.8) with extremes ranging from 18 to 55 years. The mean age of the controls was 33.6 years (standard deviation: 11) with extremes ranging from 18 to 55 years. Among patients, the typical age group was 50-55 years (25.9%). The sex ratio was 0.87 in patients and 0.99 in controls. BCG scars were present in 83.8% of TB patients and in all controls. The average number of people per room in the dwelling was 1.6 (standard deviation: 0.6), with extremes ranging from 0.4 to 4 in the patient group, and 1.5 (standard deviation: 0.7), with extremes ranging from 0.25 to 6 in the control group.

In Algeria, Amiri et al [49] conducted a descriptive retrospective study from 1[er] January 2011 to 31 December 2015 at the Annaba university hospital. The mean age of the patients was 39.05 (standard deviation: 16.74 years) with extremes ranging from 2 years to 90 years. The sex ratio was 2. This result is consistent with our study with regard to the mean age of patients.

In the French study by Delphine A and Che D [50], the median age of cases reported in 2008 was 45 years. Among patients, the average age group was 40-59 years (27.6%). The sex ratio among patients was 1.51. This is consistent with our study in terms of the modal age group of patients.

In China, according to WHO reports [51], the over-65 age group was the most represented among patients, with an M/F sex ratio of 2.1. This difference found in our study can be explained by a better hygiene of life in this country, but also by demographic reasons (ageing population in China).

In the Malian study by Rachidatou SH [52], the aim of which was to study the diameter of the TST in patients co-infected with HIV (human immunodeficiency virus) and BK (bacille de Koch), 41 subjects co-infected with tuberculosis and HIV were recruited in the country's largest hospital from 1[er] February 2006 to 28 February 2007. BCG scarring was present in 63% of subjects. This difference with the result found in our study could be explained by the inadequacy of vaccination programmes in Central African countries.

In South Korea, Lee et al [42] found that 80.7% of patients and controls had BCG scars. This result is similar to that found in our study.

In the German study by Diel et al [53], the aim of which was to study the concordance between the tuberculin TST and the ELISPOT® (Enzyme-Linked ImmunoSpot) test, an immunological test which detects latent tuberculosis infection by measuring the response to interferon γ, in a manner equivalent to the T-SPOT.TB® test [43]), in the detection of latent tuberculosis, 369 subjects were recruited from a police academy, divided into two groups according to their degree of exposure to a declared tuberculosis patient: 36 close contacts and 333 occasional contacts. The BCG scar was found in 42.8% of all contact subjects. This difference with the result of our study could be explained by the fact that the German population studied was heterogeneous, including several non-native subjects (287 subjects were born in western Germany, 74 were born in eastern Germany and 8 were born abroad).

IV.2.2. Characteristics according to the location of the tuberculosis and the induration diameter of the tuberculin TST

According to location, we found that the lymph node form represented 53.3% of all tuberculosis patients, followed by the pulmonary (35.7%) and pleural (5.6%) forms. This result differs from those found in France [50] and Algeria [49], where the pulmonary form represented 70.4% and 83.2% respectively of all tuberculosis patients. In fact, the increase in extra-pulmonary forms, and in particular the lymph node form, in Tunisia could be explained by the fact that half the cases are due to *mycobacterium bovis* and by inadequate measures to combat animal tuberculosis, an endemic disease in our population [1].

The mean diameter of the tuberculin DST induration was 13.7 mm (standard deviation: 0.7), with extremes ranging from 0 to 30 mm in patients. In controls, the mean diameter of the tuberculin DST induration was 6.2 mm (standard deviation: 6.4), with extremes ranging from 0 to 28 mm. The difference was statistically significant ($p = 10^{-6}$). In the patient group, the two modal classes of induration diameter were 10-14 mm and 15-19 mm (28.6% and 28.6% respectively). In the control group, it was 0-4 mm (45.2%).

In the German study by Diel et al [53], the mean diameter of the induration was 13.8 mm (standard deviation: 6.7) in vaccinated subjects and 16.2 mm (standard deviation: 8) in non-vaccinated subjects. This result is similar to that found in our study.

Arrad B [54] found that 6% of children with tuberculosis had an induration diameter of between 0 and 5 mm; 37.5% had an induration diameter greater than 10 mm, while 55% of TSTs were either not done or not read. This difference with our study can be explained by the fact that the study population in Morocco was infants, in whom the induration diameters were smaller.

In Mali, Rachiatou SH [52] found that 4.9% of tuberculosis patients had an induration diameter between 0 and 5 mm and 2.4% had an induration diameter greater than 10 mm. Tuberculin anergy was found in 88% of the remaining patients. The difference with our results is explained by the immune deficiencies (subjects co-infected with tuberculosis and HIV infection) at the origin of the tuberculin anergy observed.

IV.3 Estimation of indices describing the intrinsic value of a test: sensitivity, specificity and Youden index

Sensitivity and specificity are two indices of the internal validity of a test, as they do not depend on prevalence [24]. They determine the ability of the tuberculin test to differentiate between diseased and non-diseased subjects. A sensitive test is very informative when its result is negative, because it allows the physician to exclude the disease. A specific test is highly informative when the result is positive, as it enables a diagnostic hypothesis to be confirmed [21].

However, given that the results were quantitative, it was necessary to define a threshold for classifying the test results as positive or negative. For the tuberculin TST, the threshold chosen corresponded to the diameter of the induration. Calculating different sensitivity and specificity values for different induration diameters therefore necessarily involved classification errors (false positives and false negatives). Decreasing the diameter of the induration led to an increase in sensitivity (by reducing false negatives), while increasing it led to an increase in specificity (by reducing false positives). Sensitivity and specificity varied in opposite directions

[34]. This explains the limitations of sensitivity and specificity in determining the best threshold for tuberculin TST positivity in the diagnosis or screening of tuberculosis. The choice of a test's cut-off point depends on its objective. If the aim of the test is to detect the disease, it is important not to miss any cases of the condition; the positivity threshold is therefore shifted towards normal values in order to reduce false negatives and increase sensitivity. If the aim of the test is to identify a disease whose diagnosis has serious consequences (therapeutic, prognostic, psychological), it is important to confirm the diagnosis with certainty; the positivity threshold is therefore shifted towards pathological values in order to reduce false positives and increase specificity [23].

The two indices, sensitivity (Se) and specificity (Sp), are limited by the fact that they are intrinsic to the test and do not relate to the population [14]. In practice, the clinician is most often confronted with the test result rather than the status of the subject as being ill or not ill. It is therefore not possible to draw conclusions about the performance of the test on the basis of these simple concepts of sensitivity and specificity.

Other indices of the validity of the tuberculin TST can be calculated from sensitivity and specificity. These include the Youden index and likelihood ratios. The Youden index [16] is a simple synthetic index that varies between -1 and 1 and has a diagnostic orientation value. An index of 0 indicates a test that has no diagnostic value. If the index is equal to 1, the test will have maximum diagnostic value. However, the Youden index does not take into account the difference between sensitivity and specificity values. If we want to compare two tests, the first with a sensitivity of 90% and a specificity of 40% and the second with a sensitivity of 60% and a specificity of 70%, the two tests will have the same Youden index. If we refer to this index

to compare the performance of these two tests, it will therefore be wrongly concluded that the two tests have the same validity. The use of this index is therefore no longer recommended when studying the validity of diagnostic tests [55].

In our study, overall, taking age, sex and location into account, we found that for TST cut-off values > 5, 6 and 7 mm, there was no significant gain in sensitivity (the confidence intervals overlapped). There was also no significant gain in sensitivity when comparing the TST cut-off value > 7 mm with the cut-off value > 10 mm. For a cut-off value > 10 mm, sensitivity was 79.4% [95% CI: 74.7 - 83.3] and specificity was 67.6% [95% CI: 64.1 - 70.9]. For a threshold value > 11 mm, the sensitivity was 73.7% [95% CI: 68.8 - 78.1] and the specificity 76.6% [95% CI: 73.3 - 79.5]. The cut-off > 10 mm was significantly less specific than the cut-off > 11 mm (confidence intervals did not overlap), but not significantly more sensitive. When comparing the TST cut-off value > 11 mm with the cut-off value > 12 mm, there was no significant gain in sensitivity: [95% CI: 68.8 - 78.1] versus [95% CI: 64.2 - 73.9] (the confidence intervals overlapped), nor in specificity: [95% CI: 73.3 - 79.5] versus [95% CI: 76 - 81.9] (the confidence intervals overlapped).

The threshold value for the diameter of the TST > 10 mm is therefore worse than the threshold value > 11 mm. The most discriminative threshold value for the diameter of the induration of the DST, associated with the best combination of sensitivity (73.7%) and specificity (76.6%), was 11 mm with a Youden index of 0.503. We then divided the subjects into two age groups: those aged under 35 and those aged 35 and over (average age of all subjects).

For subjects aged under 35, the threshold value for the diameter of the induration of the TST, associated with the best sensitivity (79.1%) and specificity (79.8%) ratio, was 11 mm with a Youden index of 0.589.

For subjects aged 35 and over, the threshold value for the diameter of the induration of the

TST, associated with the best sensitivity (70.2%) and specificity (71.3%) ratio, was 11 mm with a Youden index of 0.415.
Depending on the location of the tuberculosis, we found that the threshold value for the diameter of the induration of the TST associated with the best {sensitivity, specificity} pair was 11 mm for both the pulmonary location (Se=70.2%; Sp=76.6%) and the lymph node location (Se=77.8%; Sp=76.6%).
In the Spanish study conducted by Altet et al [46], involving vaccinated subjects, for a TST threshold > 5mm, the sensitivity was 100% and the specificity 12%. For a tuberculin TST threshold >10mm, the sensitivity was 92% and the specificity 26%. For a tuberculin TST threshold > 15 mm, the sensitivity was 75% and the specificity 68%. The result is therefore similar to that found in our study.
In South Korea, Lee et al [42] found a sensitivity equal to 73.6% and a specificity equal to 66.4% for a threshold > 5mm. For a threshold > 10 mm, the sensitivity was 66.7% and the specificity 78.6%. For a threshold > 15 mm, the sensitivity was 43.7% and the specificity 95.4%. This result is consistent with the results of our study.
In Denmark, in the study carried out by Brock et al on unvaccinated subjects [48], for a tuberculin TST threshold > 10 mm, sensitivity was 55.5% in close contacts of tuberculosis patients and specificity was 90% in distant contacts of tuberculosis patients.
In the Netherlands, Arend et al [56] recruited 469 supermarket customers at random at the time of tuberculin TST administration and 316 with a tuberculin TST induration diameter greater than 1 mm at the time of TST reading. All subjects were unvaccinated. The aim of the study was to compare the results of the tuberculin TST, the QuantiFERON TB-Gold in Tube® and the T-SPOT.TB® in the diagnosis of tuberculosis in unvaccinated subjects. For a threshold TST > 10 mm, sensitivity was 21.4% and specificity 72% in subjects aged under 35. In subjects aged 55 and over, the sensitivity was 20.1% and the specificity 84.9%. For a threshold TST > 15 mm, the sensitivity was 18.4% and the specificity 72.2% in subjects aged under 35. In subjects aged 55 and over, the sensitivity was 24.5% and the specificity 75.3%.
The difference between the two previous studies and our results could be attributed to vaccination. In fact, cross-reactivity of the tuberculin TST with antigens of other non-tuberculous mycobacteria and with the antigen used for the BCG vaccine generates false positives leading to a false increase in sensitivity and a decrease in specificity [57, 58].
In Turkey, in the study conducted by Simsek et al [59], the aim of which was to compare the tuberculin TST and the T-SPOT.TB® in the diagnosis of latent and active tuberculosis, 136 subjects were recruited and divided into 3 groups: 47 tuberculosis patients, 47 healthy subjects and 42 healthcare workers having close contact with tuberculosis patients. Sensitivity was 83.3% and specificity 95.7% for both thresholds. This difference with the results observed in our study can also be explained by vaccination. In fact, induration diameters of between 6 and 14 mm on the tuberculin TST were attributed to the BCG vaccine. In interpreting the TST, they considered a threshold > 10 mm for unvaccinated subjects and a threshold > 15 mm for vaccinated subjects.
In the Moroccan study conducted by Arrad B [54], for a positivity threshold of 5 mm, the sensitivity was 86.5% and the specificity 88.3%. For a positivity threshold of 10 mm, the sensitivity was 84.3% and the specificity 93.5%. For a positivity threshold of 15 mm, the sensitivity was 68.5% and the specificity 97.7%. This difference with the result found in our study is probably due to the intervention of several factors such as housing, type of household, poverty and tuberculosis contagion, all of which have been shown to have a statistically significant relationship with TST positivity.

Pai et al [60], in a study published in 2008, compared the different sensitivity and specificity values of the tuberculin TST found in 38 articles worldwide.
Regardless of whether the subject was vaccinated or not, the mean sensitivity was 77% [95% CI: 71 - 82]. The mean specificity was 97% [95% CI: 95 - 99] in the unvaccinated group compared with 59% [95% CI: 46 - 73] in the vaccinated group. The thresholds considered were 5 and 10 mm respectively, depending on the study. The results found in our study are consistent with the average values calculated worldwide.

IV.4 Estimation of likelihood ratios

Likelihood ratios are validity indices used to describe the performance of a diagnostic test. They combine the information contained in the sensitivity and specificity indices. They are therefore independent of the prevalence of the disease in the population [61].
Likelihood ratios express the number of times a test result is more or less likely to be found in patients compared with nonpatients [61].
The positive likelihood ratio (LR +) represents the likelihood of obtaining a positive test in patients with the disease, compared with the likelihood of obtaining a positive test in healthy patients [18]. In clinical practice, it takes its values in the interval [1; +o>]. It quantifies the diagnostic benefit of a positive test result. The higher the positive likelihood ratio, the greater the probability that the patient has the disease [23]. In general, a positive LR > 10 is reliable and indicates that a positive test result makes a significant contribution to the diagnosis [24].
The negative likelihood ratio (LR -) represents the likelihood of obtaining a negative test in patients with the disease, compared with the likelihood of obtaining a negative test in healthy patients [18]. It takes its values in the interval [0 - 1]. It quantifies the diagnostic benefit of a negative test result. The closer the negative likelihood ratio is to 1, the lower the probability that a patient has the disease [23]. In general, a negative LR < 0.1 is reliable and indicates that a negative test result makes a significant contribution to the diagnosis [24].
Likelihood ratios are good indicators of the diagnostic value of a test. They are more useful for clinical decision-making than sensitivity and specificity. They allow the contribution of a positive (LR+) or negative (LR-) test result to be summarised in a single number [61].
They are more useful in clinical decision-making than predictive values because they are independent of prevalence and the results found could be transposable from one population to another [24].
Furthermore, likelihood ratios can be used easily and quickly to determine the positive or negative post-test probability of the disease from the a priori probability (prevalence of the disease) graphically using Fagan's nomogram [24, 36].
However, these likelihood ratios have certain limitations. Their routine use is limited by the fact that they are rarely used by practitioners, as the values of these ratios are rarely reported in epidemiological studies evaluating the performance of diagnostic tests [38].
In our study, taking age, sex and location together, we found a positive likelihood ratio of 3.1 and a negative likelihood ratio of 0.34 for a tuberculin TST threshold > 11 mm. For a threshold TST > 5 mm, the positive likelihood ratio was 1.6 and the negative likelihood ratio was 0.27. For a threshold TST > 15 mm, the positive likelihood ratio was 2.4 and the negative likelihood ratio was 0.3.
In the Spanish study by Altet et al [46], for a TST threshold > 5 mm, the positive likelihood ratio was 1.13 and the negative likelihood ratio was 0. For a threshold TST > 10 mm, the positive likelihood ratio was 1.24 and the negative likelihood ratio was 0.32. For a threshold TST >15mm, the positive likelihood ratio was 2.35 and the negative likelihood ratio was 0.37. This result is consistent with that found in our study.

In the absence of results concerning likelihood ratios in the following studies [42, 48, 54, 59], we took the liberty of calculating these indices on the basis of sensitivity and specificity for a tuberculin TST threshold > 10 mm (table X).

Table X: Positive and negative likelihood ratios in different countries calculated from the sensitivity and specificity for a tuberculin TST threshold > 10 mm.

Country	Positive likelihood ratio (LR +)	Negative likelihood ratio (LR -)
Denmark [48]	5,5	0,5
Turkey [59]	19,37	0,17
Morocco [54]	7,39	0,15
South Korea [42]	3,11	0,42
Spain [46]	1,24	0,32
Our study	**2,4**	**0,3**

Given that the calculation of likelihood ratios derives directly from sensitivity and specificity, the difference and similarity between the results can be explained by the same reasons given above. Indeed, the difference in the results found in Turkey and Denmark compared with the results found in our study can be attributed to vaccination. The intervention of several factors such as habitat, type of household, precariousness and tuberculosis contagion could explain the difference between the result found in Morocco and the result of our study. The results found in Spain and South Korea are consistent with the results of our study.

IV.5. Use of the ROC curve and estimation of the area under the curve (AUC)

IV.5.1. Use of the ROC curve

To optimise the choice of the tuberculin TST positivity threshold, we used the ROC curve and calculation of the corresponding area under the curve to measure the overall performance of the tuberculin TST.

The ROC curve was developed during the Second World War by radar technicians to distinguish between a signal from the enemy and a simple artefact [9]. It is a graphical representation of the relationship between sensitivity and specificity for all possible threshold values. It is used to determine the best discriminating threshold with the best sensitivity-specificity ratio when the test is quantitative [31, 37].

The ROC curve has several advantages [24, 25, 30, 34]:

- It is simple and easy to understand graphically;
- it takes account of all the values in the test;
- it does not depend on the prevalence of the disease in the study population, since it is based on sensitivity and specificity, both of which are independent of prevalence;
- the results provided by this curve are valid even if the sample studied is not representative;
- it allows us to set an optimal threshold that discriminates the population of patients from the population of nonpatients.

To choose the best discriminant threshold, two methods can be used based on the construction of the ROC curve. This involves calculating the square of the distance (d) separating the point (0,1) on the curve located at the apex of the upper left-hand corner from any point on the curve (possible threshold value). We write: $d^2 = (1 - \text{sensitivity})^2 * (1 - \text{specificity})^2$

The optimal threshold is the one with the lowest^2 value. The optimum threshold also corresponds to the point on the ROC curve furthest from the chance line or diagonal (Figure 27) [25, 30].

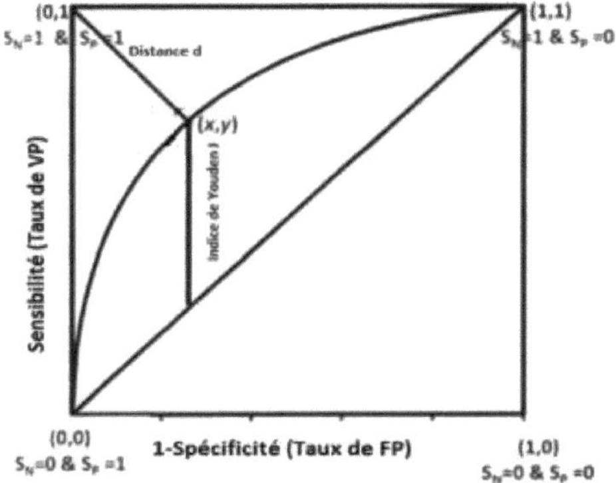

Figure 27: Example of determining the best discriminant threshold using the ROC curve.

The ROC curve also has the advantage of allowing direct visual comparison of two or more tests on the same scale [62].

Figure 28 shows two ROC curves (A and B) corresponding to two tests A and B respectively. Curve A is closer to the upper left-hand corner and therefore has a better optimum threshold than curve B. We can therefore conclude that test A performs better than test B.

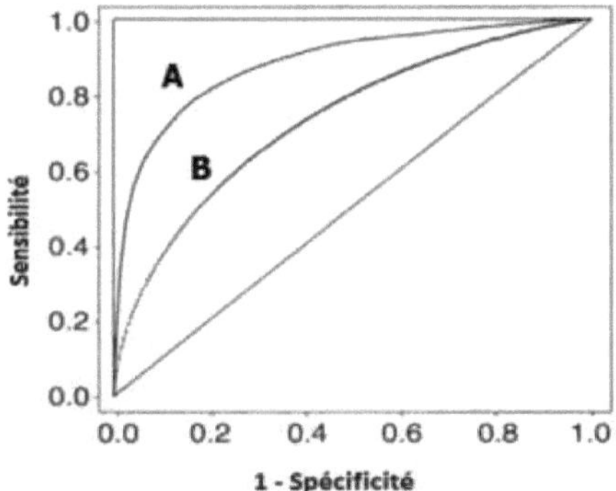

Figure 28: Example of two ROC curves A and B.

IV.5.2 Estimation of the area under the ROC curve (AUC)

After constructing the ROC curves, we calculated the corresponding areas under the curve (AUC) and their confidence intervals. We then determined the significance level p by comparing each AUC with 0.5. The area under the curve is an effective and combined measure of sensitivity and specificity that determines the validity of a diagnostic test. It varies between 0 and 1 [30].

Its advantages [25] include:

- its ability to assess the discriminatory power of a test in different situations;

- its ability to compare different ROC curves corresponding to several diagnostic tests: by comparing the area under the curve of each of them, the test with the highest AUC value is the one with the best diagnostic performance among these tests.

However, measuring the area under the curve can have certain limitations:

- Equality between the area under the curve of two tests implies that they have the same diagnostic performance but does not necessarily imply that the ROC curves of the two tests are identical [26]. This is illustrated in figure 29.

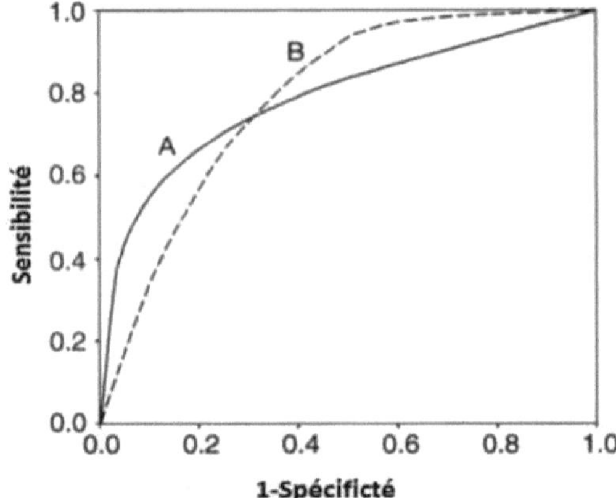

Figure 29: Example of a comparison of two ROC curves, A and B, showing the same area under the curve but a different graphical representation.

Test B is better than test A in terms of sensitivity, while test A is better in terms of specificity. Test B is therefore chosen for screening purposes (because it has the best sensitivity) and test A for diagnostic purposes (because it has the best specificity) [26].

- Calculating the area under the curve is tricky for both parametric and non-parametric shapes. If the curve is non-parametric, either the trapezoidal method [25, 26] or the non-parametric method of Hanley and Mac Neil in 1982 [33] based on the non-parametric Mann-Whitney statistic developed in 1947 [63] can be used. If the curve is parametric, the calculation is more complex and requires the use of computer programmes. In our study, we used the non-parametric method of Hanley and Mac Neil. Overall, for all ages, sexes and locations combined, the area under the AUC curve was 0.789 [95% CI: 0.758 - 0.819; p=0.01].

For the lung location, the area under the ROC curve was 0.778 [95% CI: 0.733 - 0.822; p = 0.02] while for the lymph node location, it was 0.814 [95% CI: 0.777 - 0.851; p = 0.02].

Using the ROC curve, Nayme et al [44] found that a threshold of 9 mm with a sensitivity of 68% and a specificity of 78% was sufficient for the diagnosis of tuberculosis infection, whereas a threshold of 13 mm (Se=54%; Sp=90%) was sufficient for the diagnosis of tuberculosis disease. The difference with the results found in our study is due to the high endemicity of tuberculosis in Morocco, which explains the low sensitivity values. The threshold of 13 mm was recommended, given the large number of false positives due to BCG vaccination and various latent infections with non-tuberculous mycobacteria.

IV.6. Estimation of positive and negative predictive values

In clinical practice, the most frequent situation is when a positive test is available and we want to know whether the subject is ill or not. The positive predictive value (PPV) is used to answer

this question. We therefore calculated the positive and negative predictive values (PPV and NPV) of the tuberculin TST and their confidence intervals using Bayes' theorem [35] and Fagan's nomogram [36].
The prevalence of the disease in the population studied is of considerable importance in calculating predictive values. Indeed, for a fixed sensitivity and specificity, the higher the prevalence of the disease, the higher the PPV tends towards 1 and the NPV towards 0. Conversely, the lower the prevalence, the more the PPV tends towards 0 [21].
In our study, we considered a tuberculosis prevalence level of 1% among pneumology consultants at three university hospitals in Greater Tunis. This explains the low positive predictive values reported in our study.
The calculation of predictive values also makes it possible to draw a curve representing the value of the post-test probability (equivalent to PPV, if the test result is positive, or 1-PNV if the test result is negative) as a function of the pre-test probability (equivalent to prevalence) (Figure 30).

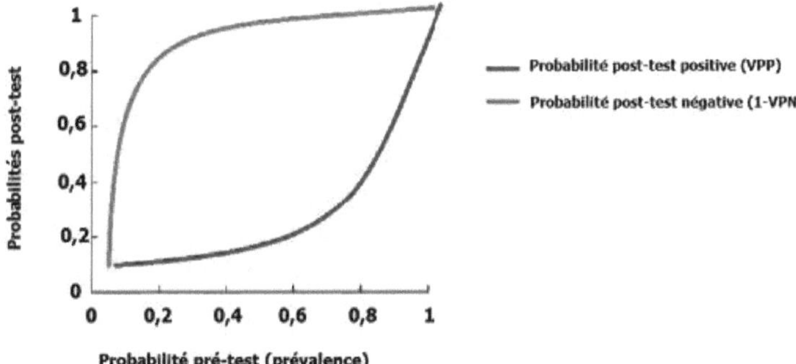

Figure 30: Variation in the positive and negative post-test probabilities as a function of the pre-test probability (prevalence).

This curve therefore shows, for any prevalence value, the gain in information provided by the test result [18]. Thus, a high prevalence implies a high positive (PPV) and negative (1-VPN) post-test probability and therefore a considerable gain in information. Conversely, a low prevalence implies a low positive and negative post-test probability and therefore a low information gain.
However, given the influence of prevalence, the predictive values observed in one study population cannot be transposed to another population where the prevalence of the disease is different. Likelihood ratios, which are independent of prevalence, are therefore increasingly used by authors [21]. Likelihood ratios help to extrapolate the performance of a test to a group of subjects different from the population in which it was studied [23].
To avoid calculating predictive values by applying Bayes' theorem, it is possible to use Fagan's nomogram, which gives the positive (PPV) and negative (1-NPV) post-test probabilities directly on a visual scale from the pre-test probability (prevalence of the disease under study) and the two positive and negative likelihood ratios [36].
This tool is very useful in clinical practice when speed is more important than precision, as it does not involve a calculator or computer. Compared with Bayes' theorem, it can be used to determine the diagnostic benefit of a positive or negative test result simply by reading the graph visually [38].
In our study, we found that for the threshold value of a tuberculin TST > 5 mm, the positive

and negative predictive values calculated using Bayes' theorem were 1.59% and 99.72% respectively, and those calculated using Fagan's nomogram were 1.7% and 99.72% respectively. For the threshold value of the tuberculin TST > 10 mm, the positive and negative predictive values calculated using Bayes' theorem were 2.4% and 99.63% respectively, and those calculated using Fagan's nomogram were 3.11% and 99.63% respectively. The two methods used therefore gave similar predictive value results.

In the Spanish study conducted by Altet et al [46], 1335 close contacts of subjects with tuberculosis were followed up for 4 years after performing a tuberculin test to predict their progression to tuberculosis disease. For a tuberculin TST induration diameter threshold > 5 mm, the positive predictive value was 2% and the negative predictive value was 100%. For a threshold TST induration diameter > 10 mm, the positive predictive value was 3% and the negative predictive value was 99%. This result is consistent with that found in our study.

In Germany, in the study conducted by Diel et al [47], 601 close contacts of subjects with tuberculosis were followed up for 103 weeks after performing a tuberculin TST in order to predict their progression to tuberculosis disease. For a threshold of positive TST > 5 mm, the positive predictive value was equal to 2.3% and the negative predictive value was equal to 99.7%. For a positive TST > 10 mm, the positive predictive value was 5.6% and the negative predictive value was 97.9%. This result is similar to that found in our study, with low positive predictive values and high negative predictive values.

In China, according to a study conducted by Leung et al [64], the aim of which was to compare the tuberculin TST and the Quantiferon T-SPOT.TB test® in the prediction of tuberculosis disease, 331 subjects with non-tuberculous silicosis recruited between 2004 and 2008 were followed up until 30 September 2009 to predict progression to tuberculosis disease.

For a threshold of positivity > 10 mm, the positive predictive value was equal to 6.6% and the negative predictive value was equal to 96.2%. The result found is consistent with the results of our study. However, the values found could be erroneous due to comorbidity bias. Subjects suffering from silicosis could be considered immunocompromised, leading to errors in the interpretation of the tuberculin TST.

Overall, using Bayes' theorem and Fagan's nomogram, taking into account the prevalence of the disease and the different validity indices of the TST (sensitivity, specificity, positive likelihood ratio and negative likelihood ratio), would provide reliable predictive value results. However, given that we only used a pre-established prevalence of tuberculosis in the population of pneumology consultants in three university hospitals in the greater Tunis area, we are unable to extrapolate the results reported in our study to the Tunisian population as a whole.

IV.7. Estimation of confidence intervals

The 95% confidence interval (CI) is an interval of values that has a 95% chance of containing the true value of the estimated parameter. With less rigour, it is possible to say that the confidence interval represents the range of values within which we are 95% certain of finding the true value we are looking for [65].

In our study, for two chosen threshold values of the tuberculin TST, and to find out whether two values of sensitivity (expressed as percentages) or two values of specificity (expressed as percentages) differ significantly at a risk of error equal to 5% (because the two proportions are subject to uncertainty) or a degree of confidence of 95%, we used another method of resolution than the comparison of two proportions on two independent samples (the equivalent of the Chi-squared test): the confidence interval approach.

The confidence interval approach thus clearly emphasises quantification, unlike p-values (degrees of significance), which are used to assess significance. The p-value is not an estimate of any quantity, but a measure of the power of the evidence in relation to the null hypothesis, reflecting the 'absence of effect'. An estimate including CIs is the best way to summarise the results of a study, but CIs and p-values are complementary, and many studies mention them both. According to this approach, if the confidence intervals of two estimates of sensitivity or specificity overlap, the two values are considered not significantly different and could represent the same true value in the population. On the other hand, if the respective confidence intervals do not overlap, then the statistical difference between the two proportions is significant [65, 66].

However, according to some authors [67, 68], this confidence interval approach is subject to certain comments. When comparing two values, if their CIs do not overlap, we can conclude that they are significantly different. On the other hand, if their CIs do overlap, the confidence interval approach does not always allow us to conclude with certainty that there is no difference between the two values being compared. In this case, it would be preferable to use the Chi-squared test or the Fischer exact test if the validity conditions of the Chi-squared test are not met [69, 70].

IV.8. Biases that may lead to erroneous estimates of the diagnostic validity criteria of the tuberculin TST

We remind you that a bias is a systematic (non-random) error introduced into the study during the selection of subjects or during the collection of information or at the time of statistical analysis. If these biases are significant, they can threaten the validity of the study. Many of these errors are difficult to detect and even more difficult to avoid [71].

We will mention a few of these which were encountered in our study and which could lead to erroneous estimates of the diagnostic validity criteria of the tuberculin TST.

In our study, the 339 sick subjects were not representative of all sick subjects in the Tunisian population, and the 714 tuberculosis-free control subjects, collected in basic health centres or district hospitals, were chosen arbitrarily and therefore not representative of all control subjects in the general population. This constituted a recruitment bias which could affect the results of our study [72].

When carrying out the tuberculin TST, the operator knew the status of the subject (sick or not sick). This could have influenced the way in which the test was performed. This was a bias measurement bias related to the operator's subjectivity, which may falsely overestimate the performance of the tuberculin TST. To control for this type of bias, the operator should evaluate the test blind to the subject's status and without clinical information [73].

The accuracy of reading an intradermal reaction, even using a rigorous technique and an experienced observer, is always limited by the variability of the test [74]. In our study, the reading of the induration diameter of the TST was performed by operators in different places and at different times, which could be a source of interpretation bias, leading to erroneous estimates of the different diagnostic validity indices of the tuberculin TST [75].

In our study, the predictive values were estimated on the basis of the prevalence of tuberculosis established in the population of pneumology consultants at three university hospitals in the greater Tunis area. These results were representative only of this population, and could not be generalised to the Tunisian population, thus constituting an extrapolation bias [76].

Our study also included an incorporation bias, as the tuberculin TST was both the test studied and part of the set of examinations used to diagnose tuberculosis [73].

Since bias is difficult to control in most cases, care must be taken to prevent its occurrence by choosing the most appropriate study design and by developing and observing rigorous protocols. In the worst case, where these biases cannot be avoided, the potential biases should at least be measured, and the possibility of statistical correction of the results should be considered [77].

IV.9. Summary and recommendations

IV.9.1. Synthesis

In our study, we evaluated the performance of the tuberculin TST through a multicentre, case-control study of adult subjects aged 18-55 years, during the period from 1er June 2014 to 30 November 2014.

We opted for this type of study because it is rapid, easy to carry out and does not require regular follow-up of the subjects surveyed. To measure the performance of the tuberculin TST, we used validity indices such as likelihood ratios, the ROC curve, the area under the ROC curve and predictive values.

Our multicentre study has shown that the tuberculin TST threshold of >11mm is the best threshold for discriminating between patients and nonpatients diagnosed with tuberculosis, regardless of age, sex or location.

For the threshold value of TST diameter > 11 mm, the positive likelihood ratio was 3.1; the negative likelihood ratio was 0.34; and the area under the ROC curve was 0.789, corresponding to moderate discriminatory power for this test.

For subjects aged under 35, the threshold value for the diameter of the induration of the TST, associated with the best sensitivity (79.1%) and specificity (79.8%) ratio, was 11 mm, with a positive likelihood ratio of 3.9 and a negative likelihood ratio of 0.26.

For subjects aged 35 and over, the threshold value for the diameter of the induration of the TST, associated with the best sensitivity (70.2%) and specificity (71.3%) ratio, was 11 mm, with a positive likelihood ratio of 2.4 and a negative likelihood ratio of 0.41.

For the pulmonary site, the threshold value for the diameter of the induration of the TST, associated with the best sensitivity (70.2%) and specificity (76.6%) ratio was 11 mm, with a positive likelihood ratio of 3 and a negative likelihood ratio of 0.39.

For lymph node location, the threshold value for the diameter of the induration of the TST, associated with the best sensitivity (77.8%) and specificity (76.6%) ratio, was 11 mm, with a positive likelihood ratio of 3.3 and a negative likelihood ratio of 0.29.

With regard to predictive values, for the threshold value > 11 mm (age, sex and location combined), the positive predictive value (PPV) and negative predictive value (NPV) calculated using Bayes' theorem were 3.11% and 99.52% respectively, and those calculated using Fagan's nomogram were 3.11% and 99.52% respectively. These predictive values, estimated on the basis of a pre-established level of tuberculosis prevalence in the population of pneumology patients attending three university hospitals in Greater Tunis, were valid only for this population.

IV.9.2 Recommendations

At the end of our study, we propose the following recommendations:

In order to estimate more precisely the various tuberculin TST evaluation indices and the thresholds of positivity for the diagnosis of tuberculosis or for the screening for tuberculosis infection, it would be interesting to carry out a prospective study which could be spread over 2 years. The sample would be made up of subjects in close contact with tuberculosis patients, recruited from anti-tuberculosis clinics, having been exposed to the tuberculosis patient for more than 6 hours a week (work colleagues, classmates, relatives, etc.). A tuberculin TST and chest X-ray will be performed on these contacts at the first visit to rule out active tuberculosis, and they will then be monitored for 2 years, with follow-up visits every 6 months. Subjects who develop the slightest symptoms of tuberculosis during this period should contact their GP immediately. They will be managed in the event of a positive diagnosis, and will then be monitored monthly during the treatment period and annually after the end of treatment. At the end of the study, contact subjects will be divided into cases and controls. Cases are subjects who have tested positive for tuberculosis during the study period. Controls will be selected at the time the case was diagnosed. They will be chosen at random from among all the controls and matched to the cases at that time. In other words, for each case diagnosed at time t, two or three controls will be chosen of the same sex, the same 5-year age group and the same duration of exposure [78]. Sensitivity and specificity are then calculated for each diameter of the tuberculin TST induration, the ROC curve and corresponding area under the curve (AUC) are derived, and likelihood ratios and predictive values are estimated. This type of study is better than the two groups of cases and controls selected at the outset, allowing control of bias and risk factors thanks to continuous follow-up of the subjects.

In order to compare the performance of the tuberculin TST and the Quantiferon test (QuantiFERON TB-Gold®) in detecting latent tuberculosis infection, it would be particularly interesting to carry out a prospective study over 2 years using the same methodology as described above. This study will be carried out on subjects in close contact with tuberculosis patients. A tuberculin TST and a Quantiferon test (appendix 5) will be carried out at the first visit. If the Quantiferon test is negative, a second test and a tuberculin TST will be repeated after 2 months. Thereafter, subjects will be monitored every 6 months for 2 years. Subjects who develop the slightest symptoms of tuberculosis should contact their GP immediately. They will be managed in the event of a positive diagnosis, and will then be monitored monthly during the treatment period and annually after the end of treatment. At the end of the study, contact subjects will be divided into cases and controls. The choice of controls will be made in the same way as in the previous study, with a degree of matching / (two controls for one case). Sensitivity and specificity will be calculated and the ROC curve and corresponding area under the curve for the tuberculin TST and the Quantiferon test respectively will be deduced. We will then compare the performance of the two tests by comparing their corresponding ROC curves. We will also compare the likelihood ratios and predictive values for the two tests.

In order to measure the performance of an established clinical score in predicting tuberculosis disease, it would be appropriate to carry out a prospective study over 2 years. The sample would be made up of close contacts of patients with tuberculosis. A tuberculin TST and a chest X-ray will be performed on these contacts at the first visit to rule out active tuberculosis, and they will then be monitored for 2 years with follow-up visits every 6 months. Subjects who develop any symptoms of tuberculosis during this study period should immediately contact the treating physician. They will be managed in the event of a positive diagnosis and will then be monitored monthly during the treatment period and annually after the end of treatment. At the end of the study, contact subjects will be divided into cases and controls. Controls will be selected in the same way as in the previous study, with a degree of matching /. A multivariate analysis of the logistic regression type [79, 80] should be performed. The factors analysed will be: age (in year classes), presence or absence of diabetes, absence of history of tuberculosis infection, absence of cough, fever lasting more than 15 days, weight loss of more than 5% and radiological appearance (normal or non-apical infiltrate without cavern, apical infiltrate without cavern, cavern or miliary). It will be necessary to ensure, on the one hand, that the variables chosen are not correlated with each other, and on the other hand, that the variables that will stand out in the analysis by having a high weight, particularly if few subjects will be concerned by this characteristic, should be considered very carefully (by performing a logarithmic transformation for example) as this could result in less accurate estimates. Thus, the relationship between each of these explanatory variables and the variable to be explained (the risk of contracting tuberculosis) will be expressed in the form of a measure of association used in epidemiology: the odds ratio (OR) and its confidence interval. The clinical score predictive of tuberculosis for each subject will be estimated as a function of the calculation of the odds ratio (OR) for each factor mentioned above [81, 82].

Next, to assess the internal validity of the clinical score, it would be interesting to carry out two other analyses on the sample in question: discrimination and calibration.

The discrimination of a score is its ability to separate subjects with and without disease for a diagnostic score [83]. This is assessed by constructing an ROC curve representing the different sensitivity values as a function of the {1-specificity} values for the different clinical scores and by calculating the area under the curve. The clinical score with the best {sensitivity, specificity} ratio will be considered the optimal score most predictive of tuberculosis disease, and the discriminatory power of this score will be considered strong if the AUC is between 0.9 and 1.

The calibration of a score makes it possible to quantify the extent to which the risk predicted by the score corresponds to the actual or observed risk. To measure the calibration, we will divide the subjects studied into ten deciles of predicted risk. For each decile, we will calculate the predicted number of subjects with tuberculosis disease by referring to the optimal clinical score established (for example, for an optimal predictive clinical score of tuberculosis > 5, subjects with a score > 5 will be considered to be ill). This stratification seems preferable to the use of threshold values fixed a priori. It makes it possible to take account of the small number of patients at the extremes. However, the overall sample must be of sufficient size, otherwise the number of strata must be reduced [83, 84].

We will then compare this predicted number with the actual number of subjects who contracted tuberculosis during the study period, using either the bar chart [83] or the Hosmer-Lemeshow test to ensure that there is no significant difference between the predicted and observed risks [85] (appendix 6).

In terms of future prospects, in order to assess external validity, it would be particularly important and interesting to determine the quality of the score on a sample other than the one from which it was developed [83, 86]. Once external validity has been established, the clinical score could be generalised to the entire population.

V CONCLUSIONS

The tuberculin skin test or intradermal reaction (IDR) to tuberculin or Mantoux test is useful both for diagnosing and screening for tuberculosis infection and for studying the delayed hypersensitivity reaction induced by BCG vaccination.
Changes in the epidemiology of tuberculosis in Tunisia (particularly the increase in the frequency of lymph node forms at the expense of pulmonary forms) have led us to reflect on the performance of the tuberculin TST in diagnosing the disease.
In the case of a test expressed by a quantitative variable, in this case the diameter of the induration of the TST, the link between the sensitivity and specificity of this test could be established very clearly.
Clearly, clinicians want a diagnostic test that is both highly sensitive and highly specific. This is not possible in practice, and a compromise must be found between sensitivity and specificity. The Receiver Operating Characteristic (ROC) curve is a way of examining the relationship between the sensitivity and specificity of the tuberculin TST.
The two characteristics, sensitivity and specificity, are intrinsic to the test and do not relate to the population. They therefore do not provide an answer to an important question for the doctor and the patient: what is the probability of being ill in the presence of a positive test (or what is the probability of not being ill in the presence of a negative test?). Likelihood ratios and positive and negative predictive values are the best indices in this case for assessing the diagnostic contribution of a positive or negative tuberculin TST result. These predictive values depend closely on the frequency of the disease (or prevalence) in the population studied.
In this study, we therefore set out to assess the performance of tuberculin TST through a multicentre, case-control study during the period from 1[er] June 2014 to 30 November 2014.
The objectives of this work were:

- to identify discriminating thresholds for the tuberculin TST test in adult subjects aged 18 to 55, using the ROC curve method in a diagnostic situation;
- determine the likelihood ratios (positive and negative) of this test;
- to determine the positive and negative predictive values of the tuberculin TST according to a pre-established level of tuberculosis prevalence.

Our study involved tuberculin intradermal testing of 339 adult patients aged between 18 and 55 years with confirmed tuberculosis, recruited at the time of the first course of anti-tuberculosis treatment in 11 tuberculosis clinics (DAT), and 714 tuberculosis-free controls, with the same sex distribution, collected in basic health centres and/or district hospitals. All the witnesses showed no respiratory or extra-respiratory signs that could be of tuberculosis origin.
A tuberculin TST data sheet has been drawn up and validated, listing the product used, the technique employed and the method for reading the diameter of the TST induration (expressed in mm).
A data collection form was filled in for each subject included in the study by the same person responsible for carrying out the tuberculin TST and reading it under the supervision of a regional coordinator.
To assess the overall performance of the tuberculin TST, we first calculated the sensitivity and specificity of the TST induration diameter and their 95% confidence intervals, as well as the Youden index for different possible thresholds (from a TST diameter > 5 mm to a TST diameter > 15 mm). We calculated the positive and negative likelihood ratios and their 95% confidence intervals, for different possible thresholds (from an RDI diameter > 5 mm to an RDI diameter > 15 mm).
We then used the ROC curve, from which we determined the most discriminative threshold

value for the diameter of the tuberculin TST induration associated with the best {sensitivity, specificity} pair. We constructed an ROC curve according to the diameter of the induration of the TST, firstly for age, sex and location combined, then according to age class and finally according to pulmonary and lymph node location. The optimal cut-off value was selected using the confidence interval approach by comparing the 95% confidence intervals of the sensitivity and specificity estimates for the tuberculin TST cut-off values chosen in pairs.

We have summarised the information contained in this curve into a simple, quantitative index, the Area Under the Curve (AUC), which has the pleasant property of summarising performance for all possible discrimination thresholds. We calculated the AUC and its 95% confidence interval, firstly for age, sex and location combined, then according to age class and finally according to lung and lymph node location. We then used a non-parametric statistic to test the area under the ROC curve against the area under the line for non-information (AUC = 0.5).

In order to estimate the informative contribution of the tuberculin TST, we calculated the positive predictive values (PPV) and negative predictive values (NPV) of the tuberculin TST and their 95% confidence intervals, for different possible thresholds (from a diameter of the TST > 5 mm to a diameter of the TST > 15 mm), age, sex and location combined. These predictive values (also called a posteriori or post-test probabilities) were estimated firstly using the properties of Bayes' theorem and secondly by establishing Fagan's nomogram, based in both cases on the prevalence of tuberculosis (also called a priori or pre-test probability) among pneumology consultants in three university hospitals in Tunis. This prevalence was estimated at around 1% in 2016.

The Fagan nomogram is a very useful tool in clinical practice when speed is more important than accuracy, because it does not involve a computer or a calculator. Compared with Bayes' theorem, it can be used to determine the diagnostic benefit of a positive or negative test result simply by reading the graph visually.

In the patient group, the mean age was 38.3 years (standard deviation: 11.8) with extremes ranging from 18 to 55 years, and the sex ratio was 0.87. In the control group, the mean age was 33.6 years (standard deviation: 11) with extremes ranging from 18 to 55 years, and the sex ratio was 0.99. BCG scarring was present in 83.8% of TB patients. It was present in all controls.

Lymph nodes accounted for 53.3% of all tuberculosis patients, followed by the lungs (35.7%) and the pleura (5.6%).

In patients, the mean diameter of the tuberculin DST induration was 13.7 mm (standard deviation: 0.7) with extremes ranging from 0 to 30 mm. In controls, the mean diameter of the tuberculin DST induration was 6.2 mm (standard deviation: 6.4) with extremes ranging from 0 to 28 mm. The difference was statistically significant (p=10).$^{-6}$

The median diameter of the induration on the tuberculin DST was 15 mm in patients and 5 mm in controls.

Regardless of age, sex and location, our study showed that the most discriminatory threshold value for the diameter of the induration of the TST, associated with the best sensitivity (73.7%) and specificity (76.6%) ratio, was 11 mm, with a Youden index of 0.503.

For the pulmonary site, the threshold value for the diameter of induration on the TST, with the best combination of sensitivity (70.2%) and specificity (76.6%), was 11 mm, with a Youden index of 0.468. For lymph node location, the threshold value for the diameter of the induration of the TST, with the best combination of sensitivity (77.8%) and specificity (76.6%), was also 11 mm with a Youden index of 0.544.

For the threshold value of 11 mm or greater (age, sex and location combined), the positive predictive value (PPV) and negative predictive value (NPV) calculated using Bayes' theorem were 3.11% and 99.52% respectively, and those calculated using Fagan's nomogram were 3.11% and 99.52% respectively. The two methods used therefore gave similar results, but were only valid for subjects consulting a respiratory clinic.

For the threshold value of the diameter of the TST greater than or equal to 11 mm, the positive likelihood ratio was equal to 3.1; the negative likelihood ratio was equal to 0.34; the area under the ROC curve was 0.789, which corresponds to moderate discriminatory power for this test.

However, our study was subject to certain biases (systematic, non-random error) which could lead to erroneous estimates of the diagnostic validity criteria for the tuberculin TST. Patient and control subjects were not representative of their respective populations, which could constitute a recruitment bias. When the tuberculin TST was performed, the operator knew the status of the subject (sick or not sick), which could have influenced the way in which the test was performed. This was a measurement bias due to the subjectivity of the operator, who could wrongly overestimate the performance of the tuberculin TST. In addition, the reading of the induration diameter of the TST was carried out by operators in different places and at different times, which could be a source of interpretation bias. In addition, the predictive values were estimated on the basis of the prevalence of tuberculosis established in the population of pneumology consultants at three university hospitals in the greater Tunis area. These results were representative only of this population, and could not be generalised to the Tunisian population, thus constituting an extrapolation bias.

At the end of our study, we propose the following recommendations:

In order to estimate more precisely the various tuberculin TST evaluation indices and the thresholds of positivity for the diagnosis of tuberculosis or for the screening of tuberculosis infection, it would be interesting to carry out a prospective study which could be spread over 2 years. The sample would be made up of subjects in close contact with tuberculosis patients, recruited from anti-tuberculosis clinics, with a duration of exposure to the tuberculosis patient of more than 6 hours per week. At the end of the study, the contact subjects will be divided into cases and controls. The sensitivity and specificity will then be calculated for each diameter of the tuberculin TST induration, the ROC curve and the corresponding area under the curve (AUC) will be derived, and the likelihood ratios and predictive values will be estimated.

In order to compare the performance of the tuberculin TST and the Quantiferon test (QuantiFERON TB-Gold®) in detecting latent tuberculosis infection, it would be particularly interesting to conduct a 2-year prospective study. This study will be carried out on subjects in close contact with tuberculosis patients. At the end of the study, the contacts will be divided into cases and controls. Sensitivity and specificity will be calculated, and the ROC curve and corresponding area under the curve for the tuberculin DST and the Quantiferon test respectively will be derived. We will then compare the performance of the two tests by comparing their corresponding ROC curves. We will also compare the likelihood ratios and predictive values for the two tests.

In order to measure the performance of an established clinical score in predicting tuberculosis disease, it would be appropriate to carry out a prospective study over 2 years. The sample would be made up of close contacts of patients with tuberculosis. At the end of the study, the contacts will be divided into cases and controls. A logistic regression type multivariate analysis should be performed. The factors analysed will be: age (in year classes), presence or absence of diabetes, absence of previous tuberculosis infection, absence of cough, fever lasting more than 15 days, weight loss of more than 5% and radiological appearance. The clinical score predictive of tuberculosis for each subject was estimated by calculating the odds ratio (OR) for each of the above factors.

Next, to assess the internal validity of the clinical score, it would be interesting to carry out two other analyses on the sample in question: discrimination and calibration.

Calibration involves comparing the predicted number of subjects with TB disease, based on the optimal clinical score, with the actual or observed risk for the groups of subjects studied, divided into ten predicted risk deciles.

In terms of future prospects, in order to assess external validity, it would be particularly important and interesting to determine the quality of the score on a sample other than the one from which it was developed. Once external validity has been established, the clinical score could be generalised to the entire population.

The establishment of clinical scores for tuberculosis could optimise the use of the various means of diagnosing tuberculosis. However, their development, validation and measurement of their clinical impact would have to meet scientific requirements, which is why collaboration between clinicians and statistical epidemiologists is essential.

Finally, ROC curves certainly have an important role to play in determining the best threshold for the tuberculin TST, making it possible to discriminate between patients who are ill and those who are not, for the diagnosis of tuberculosis or for screening for tuberculosis infection. However, it is important to emphasise the "probabilistic" nature of TST interpretation, and the fact that its predictive value can only be assessed in the light of a number of factors: epidemiological (what is the prevalence of tuberculosis?), anamnestic (is there any evidence of contact?), clinical (are there any individual risk factors?, any suggestive symptoms?) and paraclinical (favourable chest X-ray).

References

1- Ministère de la sante tunisienne, Direction des soins de sante de base, Programme national de lutte contre la tuberculose. Guide de prise en charge de la tuberculose en Tunisie, Tunis; 2014.

2- Varaine F, Henkens M, Grouzard V. Tuberculosis: A practical guide for doctors, nurses, laboratory technicians and healthcare assistants. Troisieme edition revisee. 2010.

3- Groupe de travail du Conseil Superieur d'Hygiene Publique de France. Clinical and bacteriological diagnosis of tuberculosis. Rev Mal Respir. 2003 ;20Suppl 7 :S34- S40.

4- Yombi JC, Olinga UN. TUBERCULOSIS: EPIDEMIOLOGY, CLINICAL ASPECT AND TREATMENT. Louvain Med. 2015 ;134 (10) :549-559.

5- Conseil superieur d'hygiene publique de France. Prevention and management of tuberculosis in France. Rev Mal Respir. 2003 ;20Suppl 7 :S1-S106.

6- Inserm collective expertise centre. Tuberculosis. Place de la vaccination dans la maîtrise de la maladie. 1st edition. Paris: Inserm; 2004.

7- Raising awareness of the transmission of tuberculosis through the consumption of raw milk. Livret Sante : Le magazine tunisien du mieux vivre [Online]. 2017 March [25/03/2017]; [9 pages]. Available from URL: https://livretsante.com/news/sensibilisation-tuberculose-consommation-laitcru/

8- Tunisian Ministry of Health, Directorate of Basic Health Care. Annual report on tuberculosis in Tunisia. Tunis; 2017.

9- Ben Hamida A, Mrad S, Ben Hamida L, Achour N, Zouari B, Nacef T. The diagnostic value of medical examinations: internal and predictive validity. La tunisie medicale. 1992 ;70 (4) :177-181.

10- Brown CD, Davis HT. Receiver Operating Characteristics curves and related decision measures: A tutorial. Chemometrics and Intelligent Laboratory systems. 2006 ;80 :24-38.

11- Monique Le Guen. La boite a moustaches pour sensibiliser a la statistique. Bulletin de Methodologie Sociologique / Bulletin of SociologicalMethodology. 2002 ;73 (1) :43- 64.

12- Monique Le Guen. The TUKEY moustache box, a tool to introduce you to Statistics. Statistiquement Votre - SFDS. 2001 :1-3.

13- Excel calculator reference

14- Mancini J, Gaudart J, Giorgi R. Criteria for evaluating the performance and utility of a diagnostic test. Med Trop. 2009;69 :78-82.

15- Nendaz MR, Perrier A. Sensitivity, specificity, positive predictive value and negative predictive value of a diagnostic test. Rev Mal Respir. 2004 ;21 :390-3.

16- McCluskey BSc A, Lalkhen AG. Clinical tests: sensitivity and specificity. Continuing Education in Anesthesia, Critical Care and Pain. 2008 ;8(6) :221-223.

17- Youden WJ. An index for rating diagnostic test. American Cancer Society. 1950 ;3 :32-5.

18- Jean-Marc Daigle. L'utilisation des courbes ROC dans l'évaluation des tests diagnostiques de laboratoire clinique : Application a l'etude de la pneumonie d'hypersensibilite [These]. Departement de mathematiques et de statistique : Laval ; 2002. 72 p.

19- Colombet I, Touze E. Diagnostic performance indices. Sang Thrombose Vaisseaux. 2011 ;23 (6) :307-16.

20- Akobeng AK. Understanding diagnostic tests 2: likelihood ratios, pre- and post-test probabilities and their use in clinical practice. Acta Paediatrica. 2006;96 :487-491.

21- Goeldin AO, Perrig M. Evidence-based clinical examination. Primary and hospital

care - Medecine interne generale. 2016 ;16(6) :109-112.
22- Quenet S, Presles E, Le Gal G. Evaluation des examens diagnostiques. mt. 2005 ;11(5) :318-323.
23- Nendaz MR, Perrier A. Bayes' theorem and likelihood ratios. Rev Mal Respir. 2004 ;21 :394-7.
24- Delacour H, ServonnetA , Perrot A, Vigezzi JF, Ramirez JM. The ROC curve: principles and main applications in clinical biology. Ann Biol Clin. 2005 ;63(2) :145-54.
25- Delacour H, Servonnet A, Roche C. Criteria for evaluating the validity of a biological test. Revue Francophone des Laboratoires. 2009 ; (412) :41-48.
26- Delacour H, Francois N, Servonnet A, Gentile A, Roche B. Likelihood ratios: a tool of choice for the interpretation of biological tests. Immunoanalyse et biologie specialisee. 2009 ;24 :92-99.
27- Kumar R, Indrayan A. Receiver Operating Characteristic Curve for Medical Researchers. INDIAN PEDIATRICS. 2011 ;48 : 277-87.
28- Park SH, Goo JM , Jo CH : Receiver Operating Characteristic Curve: Practical Review for Radiologists. Korean J Radiol. 2004 ;5 :11-18.
29- Althouse AD. Statistical Graphics in action: making better sense of the ROC curve. International Journal of Cardiology. 2016 ;215 :9-10.
30- Morin V, Morin JF, Mercier M, Moineau MP, Codet JP. ROC curves in medical biology (ClockAround the ROC). ImmunoanalBiolSpec. 1998 ;13 :279-286.
31- Hannequin P, Liehn JC, Deltour G. Utilisation des courbes ROC pour l'interprétation des dosages biologiques : application au dosage radio-immunologique de la thyroglobuline. Trait d'Union. (6) :31-36.
32- Hajian-Tilaki K. Receiver Operating Characteristic Curve Analysis for Medical Diagnotic Test Evaluation.Caspian J Intern Med. 2013 ;4 (2) :627-635.
33- Perneger T, Perrier A. Analysis of a diagnostic test: receiver operating characteristic (ROC) curve. Rev Mal Respir. 2004 ;21 :398-401.
34- Daya S. Diagnostic test - receiver operating characteristic (ROC) curve. Evidence-based Obstetrics and Gynecology. 2006; 8 :3-4.
35- Hanley J A MBJ. The meaning and use of the area under a receiver operating charcteristic(ROC) curve. Radiology. 1982 ;143:29-36.
36- Reference Epi-Info
37- Boyer P. Understanding diagnostic tests. Gazette de l'AFAR. 2013 ; (78) :14-20.
38- Bayes T. An essay toward solving a problem in the doctrine of chances. Philos Trans R SocLond. 1763 ;53 :370-418.
39- Fagan TJ. Nomogram for Bayes theorem. N eng J med. 1975 ;293:257.
40- Caraguel CGB, Vanderstichel R. The two-step Fagan's nomogram : ad hoc interpretation of a diagnostic test result without calculation. Evid Based Med. 2013;18 (4) :125-28.
41- Reference on the application of the Fagan nomogram
42- Working group of the Conseil Superieur d'Hygiene Publique de France. Intradermal tuberculin reaction (TDR) or tuberculin test. Rev Mal Respir. 2003 ;20Suppl 7 :S27-S33.
43- Foundation against respiratory diseases and for health education. Recommendations for target screening and treatment of latent tuberculosis infection. Brussels; 2003.
44- Lee JY, Choi HJ, Park IN, Hong SB, Oh YM, Lim CM et al. Comparison of two commercial interferon-Gamma assays for diagnosing Mycobacterium tuberculosis infection.

EurRespir J. 2006 ;28 :24-30.
45- Conseil superieur d'hygiène de France Section des Maladies Transmissibles. The Diagnosis of latent tuberculosis infection using INTERFERON-GAMMA release assays (IGRAs). Recommendation for clinical practice. June 2011.
46- Nayme I, Soualhi M, Idahmed I, Jniene A, Zahraoui R, Iraqui G. Test de Mantoux :
What threshold? EasternMediterraneanHealth Journal. 2012 ;18 (8) :870- 74.
47- Mori T, Sakatani M, Yamagishi F, Takashima T, Kawabe Y, Nagao K et al. Specific Detection of Tuberculosis Infection An Interferon--based Assay Using New Antigens. Am J RespirCrit Care Med. 2004 ;170 :59-64.
48- Altet N, Dominguez J, de Souza-Galvao ML, Angeles Jimenez-Fuentes M, Mila C, Solsona J et al. Predicting the Development of Tuberculosis with the Tuberculin Skin Test and QuantiFERON Testing. Ann Am Thorac Soc. 2015 ;12(5) :680 - 88.
49- Diel R, Loddenkemper R, Meywald-Walter K, Nieman S, Nienhaus A. Predictive Value
of a Whole Blood IFN-g Assay for the Development of Active Tuberculosis Disease after Recent Infection with Mycobacterium tuberculosis. Am J RespirCrit Care Med. 2008 ;177 :1164-70.
50- Brock I, Weldingh K, Lillebaek T, Follmann F, Andersen P.Comparison of Tuberculin Skin Test and New Specific Blood Test in Tuberculosis Contacts. Am J RespirCrit Care Med. 2004 ;170 :65 - 69.
51- Amiri S, Amoura K, Bouaricha A, Nedjai S, Benali A, Dekhil M : Frequence de la tuberculose au CHU- Annaba. Revue Tunisienne d'Infectiologie. 2016 ;10Suppl 1 :S1- S135.
52- Delphine A, Che D. Epidemiology of tuberculosis in France: a review of cases declared in 2008. Weekly epidemiological bulletin. 2010 ; (27-28) :289-293
53- WHO Global Tuberculosis Control Report 2015.
54- Rachidatou SH. Study of the tuberculin intradermoreaction in patients with tuberculosis.
atteints de tuberculose et de SIDA au CHU du point G [These]. Faculte de medecine, de pharmacie et d'odonto-stomatologie: Bamako; 2008. 110 p.
55- Diel R, Ernst M, Doscher G, Visuri-Karbe L, Greinert U, Niemann S. Avoiding the effect of BCG vaccination in detecting Mycobacterium tuberculosis infection with a blood test. EurRespir J. 2006 ; 28 :16-23.
56- Arrad B. Interpretation of the tuberculin intradermoreaction in children of age scolaire de la prefecture de Marrakech [These]. Universite CADI AYYAD Faculte de medecine et de pharmacie : Marrakech ; 2010. 65 p.
57- Ana-Maria Simundic. Measures of Diagnostic Accuracy: Basic Definitions. EJIFCC. 2009 ;19(4) : 203-211.
58- Arend SM, Thijsen SFT, Leyten EMS, Bouwman JJM, Franken WPJ, Koster BFPJ et al.
Comparison of Two Interferon-Assays and Tuberculin Skin Test for Tracing Tuberculosis Contacts. Am J RespirCrit Care Med. 2007 ;175 :618-27.
59- Tissot F, Zanetti G, Francioli P, Zellweger JP, Zysset F. Influence of BacilleCalmette-Guerin Vaccination on Size of Tuberculin Skin Test Reaction: To What Size? CID. 2005 ;40 :211-217.
60- Lee E, Holzman RS. Evolution and Current Use of Tuberculin Test. CID. 2002; (34) :365-70.
61- Simsek H, Alpar S, U^ar N, Aksu F, Ceyhan I, Gozalan A et al. Comparison of

Tuberculin Skin Testing and T-SPOT TB for Diagnosis of Latent and Active Tuberculosis. Jpn. J. Infect. Dis. 2010 ;63 : 99-102.
62- Pai M, Zwerling A, Menzies D. Systematic Review: T-Cell-based Assays for the Diagnosis of Latent Tuberculosis Infection: An Update. Ann Intern Med. 2008 ;149 (3) :177-184.
63- Fletcher RH, Fletcher SW, Wagner EH. Clinical Epidemiology. 3rd edition. Paris: Pradel; 1998.
64- Moise A, Salamon R, Commenges D, Clement B. The use of ROC curves. Rev. Epidem. et Sante Publ. 1986; 34: 209-217.
65- Faraggi D RB. Estimating of area under the ROC curve. Stat Med. 2002 ;21 :3093-3106.
66- Leung CC, Yam WC, Yew WW, Ho PL, Tam CM, Law WS et al. T-Spot.TB Outperforms Tuberculin Skin Test in Predicting Tuberculosis Disease. Am J RespirCrit Care Med. 2010 ;182 :834-840.
67- Melot C: What is a confidence interval. Rev Mal Respir. 2003; 20:599-601.
68- Braitman LE. Confidence Intervals Assess Both Clinical Significance and Statistical Significance. Annals of Internal Medicine. 1991 ;114(6) : 515-517.
69- Cole SR, Cliff Blair R. Overlapping confidence intervals. J AM ACAD Dermatol. 1999; 41(6) :1051-52.
70- Austin PC, Hux JE. A brief note on overlapping confidence intervals. J VascSurg. 2002
;36(1) : 194-5.
71- Vallee Polneau S, DIAINE C. COMPARISON OF FISHER'S EXACT TEST AND CHI-SQUARE APPLIED TO CONTINGENCY TABLES WITH TWO ROWS AND TWO COLUMNS. Cah. Sante Publique. 2015 ;14(1) :55-62.
72- McHugh ML. The Chi-square test of independence. BiochemiaMedica. 2013 ;23(2) :143-9.
73- Touzet S., Chapuis F, Colin C. Aspects methodologiques de l'évaluation du depistage
About screening for viral hepatitis C. Gastroenterol Clin Biol. 2000 ;24 :631- 36.
74- Ranque B, Mechtouff L, Grabar S. Epidemiology and etiology: from risk factor to risk outcome.
the cause. Sang Thrombose Vaisseaux. 2011 ; 23(5) :242-52.
75- Watine J. Revue systematique et meta-analyses en biologie clinique : principes et methods. Ann Biol Clin. 2004 ;62 :611-27.
76- Bierrenbach AL et al. A comparison of dual skin test with Mycobacterial antigens and
tuberculin skin test alone in estimating prevalence of Mycobacterium tuberculosis infection in a population survey. International Journal of Tuberculosis and Lung Disease. 2003 ;7 :312-319.
77- Albert-Charpentier S. Evaluation of Biological Diagnostic Tests
d'Evenements Coronariens Aigus en Medecine d'Urgence [These]. Epidemiology, Toulouse 3 Paul Sabatier University; 2010. 200 p.
78- Michiels B, Eerstelijns V. The advantages and disadvantages of case-control studies on a sample. Minerva. 2016 ;15 (4) :105-106.
79- WORLD HEALTH ORGANISATION Western Pacific Regional Office
Manila, 2003, METHODOLOGIE DE LA RECHERCHE DANS LE DOMAINE DE LA SANTE Guide

de formation aux methodes de la recherche scientifique, Second edition.
80- Nowak E, Oger E, Mottier D. Observational studies: case-control and cohort. Mt. 2008 ;14 (1) :37-46.
81- Preux PM, Odermatt P, Perna A, Marin B, Vergnenegre A. What is a
Rev Mal Respir. 2005 ;22: 159-62.
82- El Sanharawi M, Naudet F. Comprendre la regression logistique. Journal fran^ais of ophthalmology. 2013 ;36 :710-715.
83- Guessous I, Durieux-Paillard S. Validation des scores cliniques : notions theoriques et
basic practices. Rev Med Suisse. 2010 ;6 :1798-802.
84- Gauthier E. Assessing the risk of disease: designing a process and an information system allowing the construction of a risk score adapted to the context, application to breast cancer [These]. Telecom Bretagne, Universite de Bretagne-Sud; 2013. 188 p.
85- Hosmer DW, Lemeshow S. A goodness-of-fit test for the multiple logistic regression model. Comm Stat. 1980; 10 :1043-1069.
86- Kone A, Horo K, Koffi M, Samake K, Ahui B, Brou-Gode C et al. Diagnostic score of pulmonary tuberculosis in endemic tuberculosis areas. Rev Mal Respir. January 2016 ;33Suppl :A157.
87- Haut Conseil de la Sante Publique, Commission specialisee Maladies transmissibles. Tuberculosis and interferon gamma detection tests. 1st July 2011.
88- Delory T. Development of a predictive model for pulmonary tuberculosis in a group of patients.
patients suspected of having tuberculosis in a low-prevalence area: a case-control study [These]. Medecine humaine et pathologie : Paris ; 2015. 32p.

Appendices

Appendix 1
Data collection form

Survey date: /__/_//_/_//_/_/_/_/_/_/
Region: ....
DAT number :
Patient with confirmed tuberculosis /__/_____ / Patient free of tuberculosis /__/
Place of recruitment of the patient free of tuberculosis :
CSB /__/ District hospital //
Age (year) : /__/__/
Sex: M /__/F /__/
Niveau d'instruction : Analphabete //Primaire //Secondaire //Superieure //
Presence of vaccine scar : *1 /__/ yes ; 2 /__ / no*
Patient already treated for pulmonary or extra-pulmonary TBC: *1 /__/yes 2/__ / no*
- Subject with a pathological condition that may lead to tuberculin anergy:
- acute viroses (measles, mumps, infectious mononucleosis, influenza): *1 /_______ / yes ; 2 ________________ /_/no*
- lymphoma : *1 /__/ yes ; 2 /__ no*
- neoplastic pathology : *1 /__/ yes ; 2 /__ / no*
- sarcoidosis : *1 /__/ yes ; 2 /__/ no*
- severe bacterial infection : *1 /__/ yes ; 2 /__ no*
- HIV infection : *1 /__/ yes ; 2 /__ / no*
- Subject (patient or witness) with :
  immunosuppressive treatment: *1 /__/ yes; 2 /__ no*
  a corticotherapie since more than one month: *1 /__/ yes; 2 /__ no*
- or a vaccination with live attenuated vaccines two months prior to the test:

1 /__/ yes ; 2 /__ / no
- Subjects (patients or bystanders) with a history of known allergic reaction to one of the components of tuberculin or during previous administration
1 /__/ yes ; 2 /__ / no
Patient: location of tuberculosis :..
IDR :
Date de realisation : /__/__/ /__/__/ /__/__/__/__/
Diameter of induration (mm) : /_//
Associated reactions: erythema /__/ phlyctene /__/ necrosis /__/ lymphangitis /__/

Appendix 2
Technical sheet on the tuberculin test

Material -The tuberculin available is: **PPD RT 23 SSI tuberculin** from Statens Serum **Necessary:** Institute of Denmark.
Vials of 10 doses (of 0.1ml each) to be stored at a temperature of between 2°C and 8°C in the original packaging to protect the product from light. Use within 24 hours of the first opening of the vial - A fine, short (1cm) intradermal needle with a short bevel and a 1ml graduated syringe with a leak-proof plunger - Alcohol or ether and cotton wool - A transparent graduated ruler

Technique injection: After simple cleansing of the skin with alcohol or ether at the injection site The person carrying out the test grasps the forearm with his or her full hand in order to stretch it out as far as possible.

the skin, then injects with the other hand, **inserting the needle tangentially into the dermis** as soon as the upper part of the bevel has disappeared into the skin the tuberculin is injected slowly, watching the stroke of the plunger between the graduations on the syringe to ensure that exactly **0.1 ml** of tuberculin is injected.

The injection of 0.1ml of tuberculin solution must be made strictly intradermally on the front of the forearm at the junction of the upper third and the lower two thirds of the forearm, at a distance from any scars.

If the intradermal injection has been carried out correctly, the product is difficult to inject and **a white, raised dermal papule** forms around the tip of the needle, **giving an "orange peel" appearance.** If this papule does not appear, the needle is not inside the dermis: the needle must be removed and a new injection made.

It is **read** 72 hours after the injection and involves observing the reaction on the **test :** the skin and measuring the reaction.

*Observation of the skin at the injection site shows different aspects:

- or the skin is normal
- or it is covered by a more or less red papule in the centre. This papule is sometimes surrounded by a large red areola or surmounted by a few phlyctenes.
- The test result must be measured accurately: **palpation of the reaction is used to identify the indurated outline of the papule** (not the redness), which is marked with a pen. The transverse diameter of the induration (not its vertical diameter) is then measured using a transparent ruler. The test result is always expressed in millimetres.

Appendix 3

Box-Plot or moustache box

The TUKEY box-plot is a representation of a statistical series used to describe the distribution of a quantitative variable by incorporating central tendency and dispersion parameters [11, 12]. The parameters making up the Box-Plot include :

- The scale of values for the variable, located on the vertical axis
- There are three quartiles (positional parameters) to divide up the distribution into four equal parts.

> The first quartile (Q_1: 25eme percentile): separates 25% of the lowest values and 75% of the highest values.

> The second quartile (Q_2) or median: separates the distribution into 2 equal parts

> The third quartile (Q3: 75eme percentile): separates 75% of the lowest values and 25% of the highest values.

- The interquartile range (IQ) (dispersion parameters), which corresponds to 50% of observations in the central part of the distribution, is equivalent to $Q_3 - Q_1$.
- The top and bottom whiskers are represented by small vertical rectangles on either side of the box.
- The two adjacent values delimiting the upper and lower whiskers

> The minimum adjacent value corresponds to the value in the series that is immediately greater than the low border value, which is equal to : $Q_1 - 1.5 * IQ$

> The maximum adjacent value corresponds to the value of the series immediately below the high border value, which is equal to : $Q_3 + 1.5 * IQ$

- The average is sometimes shown as a cross (x)
- The so-called extreme or atypical values, also called "outliers", are located beyond the adjacent values. They are represented by markers (squares, stars, etc.).

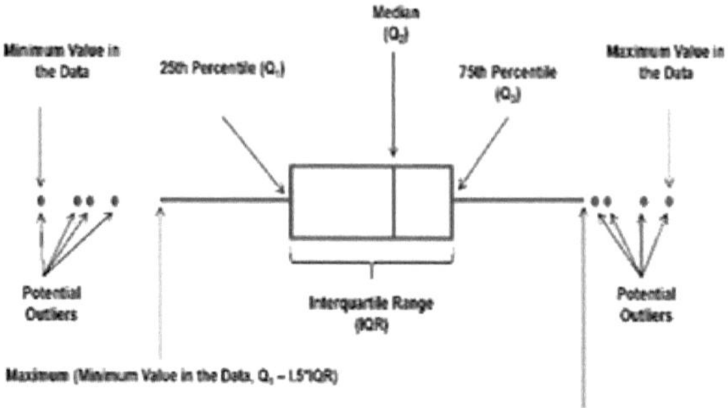
Median (Q2)
Minimum Value in the Data
25th Percentile (Q1)
75th Percentile (Q3)
Maximum Value in the Data
Potential Outliers
Interquartile Range (IQR)
Potential Outliers
Maximum (Minimum Value in the Data, Q1 – 1.5*IQR)
Minimum (Maximum Value in the Data, Q3 + 1.5*IQR)

.

Appendix 4
Fagan nomograms
for different critical thresholds of the tuberculin TST
age, gender and location combined

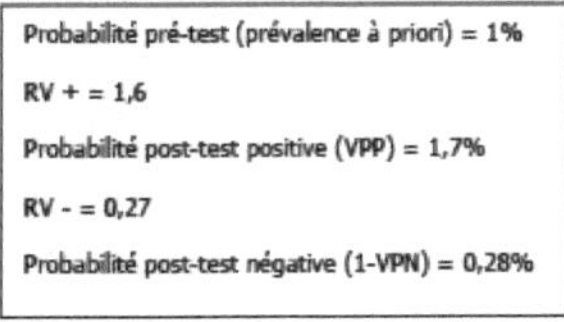

Probabilité pré-test (prévalence à priori) = 1%

RV + = 1,6

Probabilité post-test positive (VPP) = 1,7%

RV - = 0,27

Probabilité post-test négative (1-VPN) = 0,28%

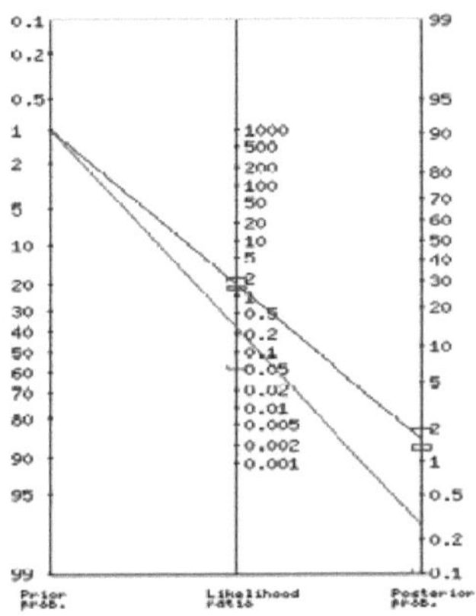

Probability pre-test (prevalence a priori) = 1%
RV + = 1.6
Probability post-test positive (PPV) = 1.7
RV - = 0.27
Probability post-test negative (1-VPN) = 0.28

Figure 17: Fagan nomogram
for a critical threshold for tuberculin TST > 5 mm.

Probabilité pré-test (prévalence à priori) = 1%

RV + = 1,7

Probabilité post-test positive (VPP) = 1,86%

RV - = 0,27

Probabilité post-test négative (1-VPN) = 0,25%

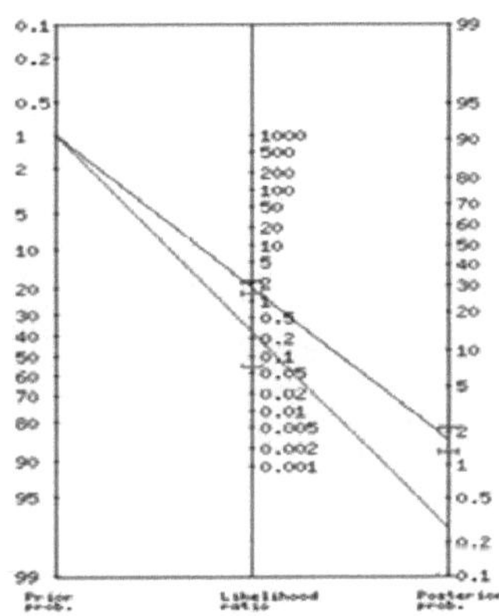

Pre-test probability (a priori prevalence) = 1%.
RV + = 1.7
Probability post-test positive (PPV) = 1.86%.
RV - = 0.27
Probability post-test negative (1-VPN) = 0.25

Figure 18: Fagan nomogram
for a critical threshold of tuberculin TST > 6 mm.

Probabilité pré-test (prévalence à priori) = 1

RV + = 1,9

Probabilité post-test positive (VPP) = 1,81%

RV - = 0,27

Probabilité post-test négative (1-VPN) = 0,2

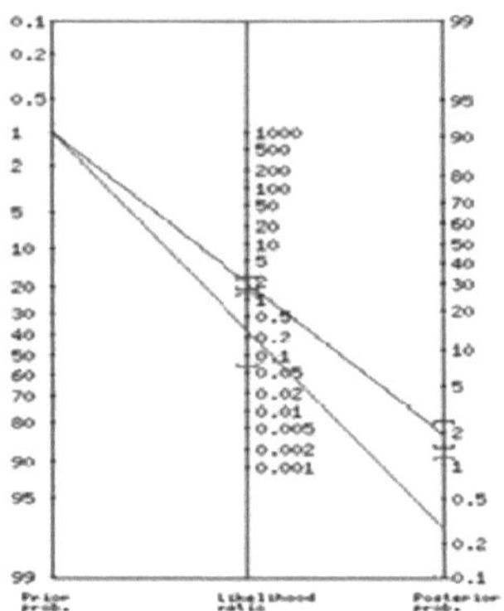

Probability pre-test (prevalence a priori) = 1
RV + = 1.9
Positive post-test probability (PPV) = 1.81%.
RV - = 0.27
Probability of negative post-test (1-VPN) = 0.2:

Figure 19: Fagan nomogram
for a critical threshold of tuberculin RDI > 7 mm.

Probabilité pré-test (prévalence à priori) = 1%

RV + = 2

Probabilité post-test positive (VPP) = 2,02%

RV - = 0,27

Probabilité post-test négative (1-VPN) = 0,22%

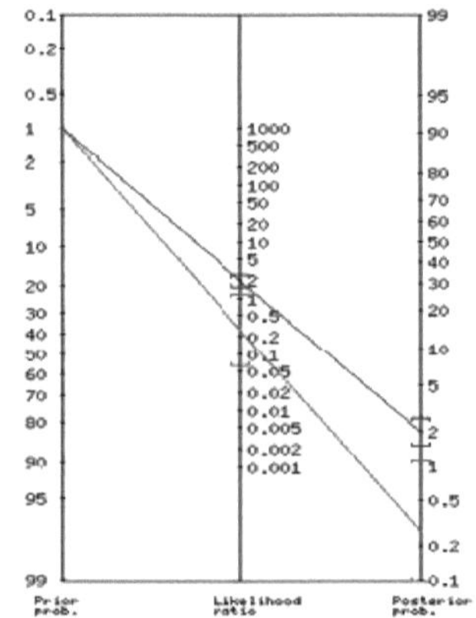

Pre-test probability (a priori prevalence) = 1%.
RV + = 2
Positive post-test probability (PPV) = 2.02%.
RV - = 0.27
Probability of negative post-test (1-VPN) = 0.22

Figure 20: Fagan nomogram
for a critical threshold for tuberculin TST > 8 mm.

Probabilité pré-test (prévalence à priori) = 1%

RV + = 2,3

Probabilité post-test positive (VPP) = 2,07%

RV - = 0,29

Probabilité post-test négative (1-VPN) = 0,39%

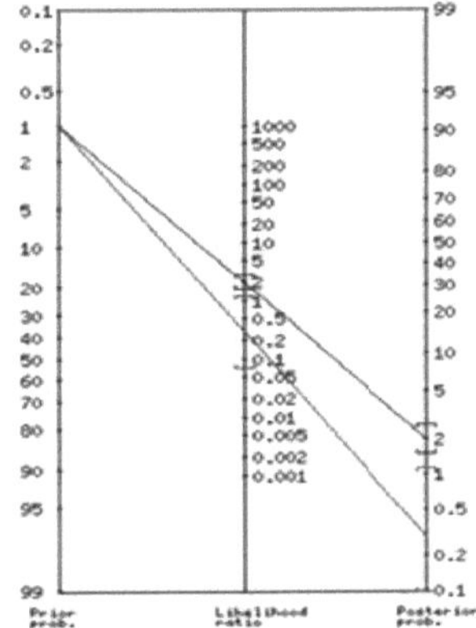

Pre-test probability (a priori prevalence) = 1%.
RV + = 2,3
Positive post-test probability (PPV) = 2.07%.
RV - = 0.29
Probability of negative post-test (1-VPN) = 0.39%.

Figure 21: Fagan nomogram
for a critical threshold of the tuberculin TST > 9 mm.

Probabilité pré-test (prévalence à priori) = 1%

RV + = 2,4

Probabilité post-test positive (VPP) = 2%

RV - = 0,3

Probabilité post-test négative (1-VPN) = 0,37%

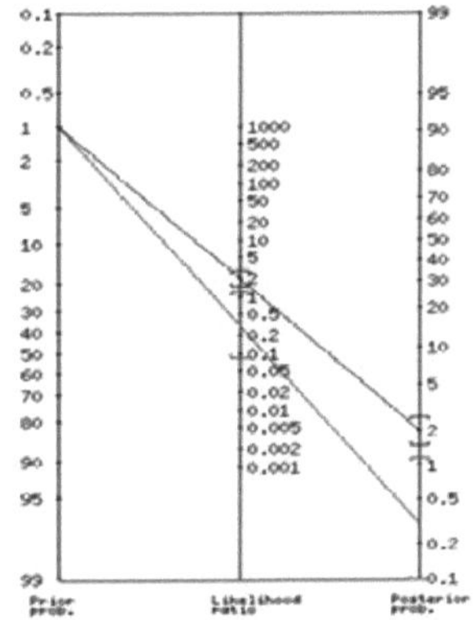

Pre-test probability (a priori prevalence) = 1%.
RV + = 2.4
Probability post-test positive (PPV) = 2%.
RV - = 0.3
Probability post-test negative (1-VPN) = 0.37

Figure 22: Fagan nomogram
for a critical threshold for tuberculin TST > 10 mm.

Probabilité pré-test (prévalence à priori) = 1%

RV + = 3,3

Probabilité post-test positive (VPP) = 3,38%

RV - = 0,39

Probabilité post-test négative (1-VPN) = 0,45%

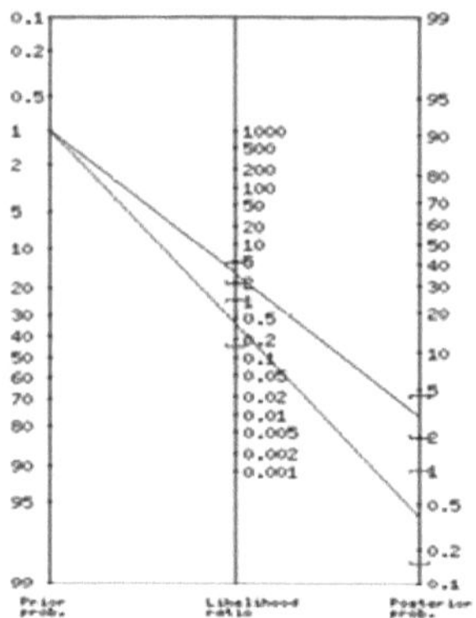

Probability pre-test (prevalence a priori) = 1%
RV + = 3.3
Positive post-test probability (PPV) = 3.38%.
RV - = 0.39
Probability of negative post-test (1-VPN) = 0.45%.

Figure 23: Fagan nomogram
for a critical threshold of the tuberculin TST > 12 mm.

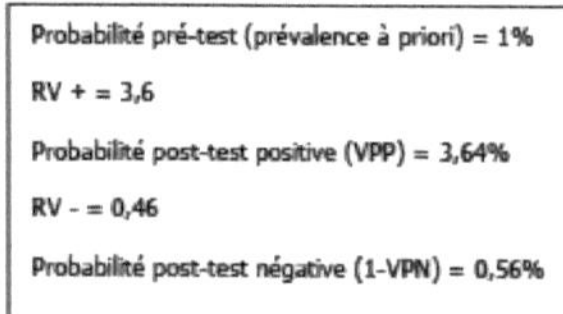

Probabilité pré-test (prévalence à priori) = 1%

RV + = 3,6

Probabilité post-test positive (VPP) = 3,64%

RV - = 0,46

Probabilité post-test négative (1-VPN) = 0,56%

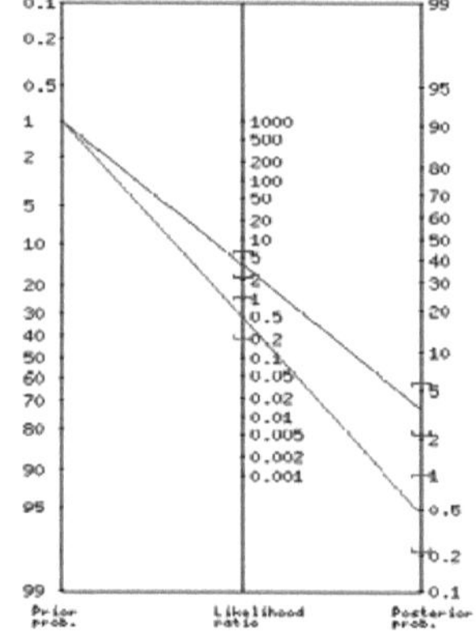

Pre-test probability (a priori prevalence) = 1%.
RV + = 3.6
Positive post-test probability (PPV) = 3.64%.
RV - = 0.46
Probability of negative post-test (1-VPN) = 0.56%.

Figure 24: Fagan nomogram
for a critical threshold of the tuberculin TST > 13 mm.

Probabilité pré-test (prévalence à priori) = 1%

RV + = 4,1

Probabilité post-test positive(VPP) = 4,25%

RV - = 0,52

Probabilité post-test négative (1-VPN) = 0,52%

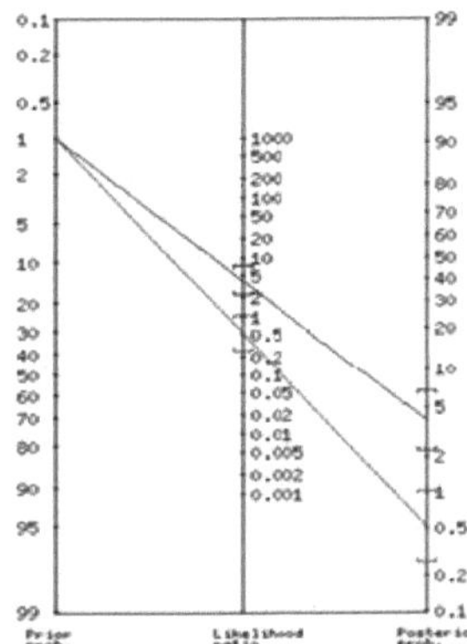

Pre-test probability (a priori prevalence) = 1%.
RV + = 4.1
Positive post-test probability (PPV) = 4.25%.
RV - = 0.52
Probability of negative post-test (1-VPN) = 0.52

Figure 25: Fagan nomogram
for a critical threshold of the tuberculin TST > 14 mm.

Probabilité pré-test (prévalence à priori) = 1%

RV + = 4,4

Probabilité post-test positive (VPP) = 4,31%

RV - = 0,56

Probabilité post-test négative (1-VPN) = 0,63%

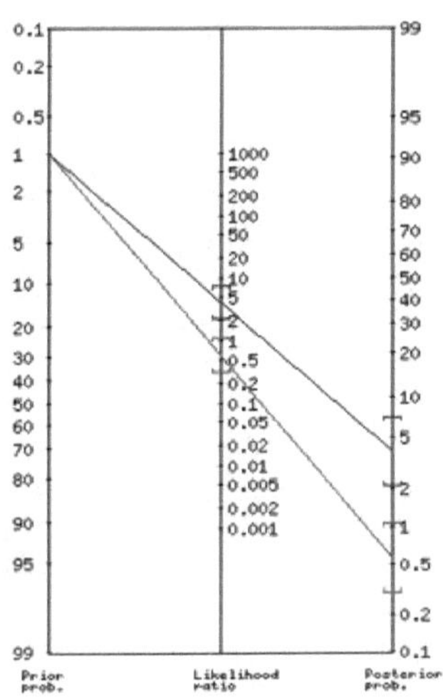

Probability pre-test (prevalence a priori) = 1%
RV + = 4.4
Probability post-test positive (PPV) = 4.31%.
RV - = 0.56
Probability of post-test negative (1-VPN) = 0.63%.

Figure 26: Fagan nomogram
for a critical threshold of the tuberculin TST > 15 mm.

Appendix 5
Technical data for QuantiFERON TB-Gold in Tube®
used in Tunisia

QuantiFERON TB-Gold in Tube® measures an immunological response (interferon gamma response) and is an alternative to the tuberculin TST for detecting latent tuberculosis infection. In this test, synthetic peptides (ESAT-6, CFP-10 and Tb 7,7 peptide) with a high degree of structural homology with *M.Tuberculosis* proteins are used, which are more specific for the Koch bacillus than the standardised tuberculin used for the tuberculin TST. Detection of interferon-Y (IFN-Y) by enzyme-linked immunosorbent assay (ELISA) is used to identify in vitro responses to peptide antigens associated with infection by *Mycobacterium tuberculosis* [45]. This test is very expensive (100 dinars in the public sector and around 210 DT in the private sector) compared with the tuberculin TST, which is free.

To carry out the QuantiFERON TB-Gold in Tube test® , the following procedures must be followed: For each subject, draw 1 ml of blood by venipuncture directly into each QuantiFERON TB-Gold in Tube® collection tube. These tubes include a zero value tube, a TB antigen tube and a mitogen tube.

1. Immediately after filling the tubes, shake them ten (10) times hard enough to ensure that the entire inner wall of the tube is lined with blood, in order to dissolve any antigen present on the walls of the tube.
2. Label the tubes correctly.
3. After filling, shaking and labelling, the tubes should be transferred to an incubator at 37°C ± 1°C as soon as possible and within 16 hours of collection. Prior to incubation, tubes should be maintained at room temperature (22°C ± 5°C). Do not refrigerate or freeze blood samples.
4. After an incubation period of 16 to 24 hours, the tubes are centrifuged, the plasma is removed and the amount of IFN-y (IU/ml) is measured by ELISA. A test is considered positive if the IFN-y response to the TB antigen tube is significantly greater than the IFN-y cut-off value (the cut-off value recommended by the manufacturer and used in various studies [49, 50] is 0.35 IU/ml).

Appendix 6
Measuring the calibration of a clinical score

- The bar chart is the most commonly used graphical representation for measuring the calibration of a clinical score. On the abscissa, the predicted risk is plotted in ten equal categories. On the ordinate, we plot the risk predicted by the clinical score and the observed or actual risk for each of the ten groups. If, for each group, the bars representing the predicted number of sick subjects are close to the bars representing the actual or observed number, and if the size of the bars increases with the groups or deciles, the score is well calibrated [83].

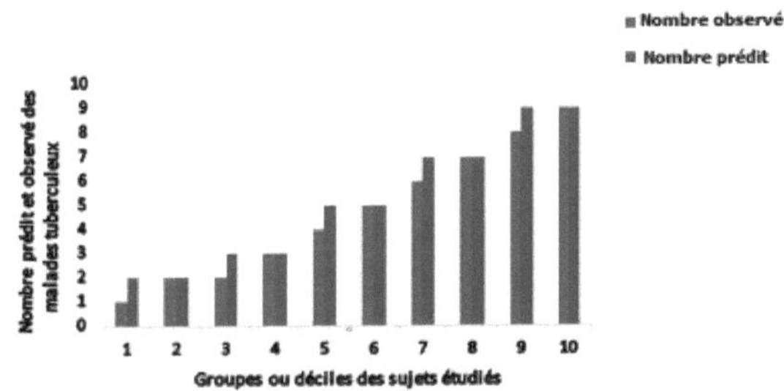

Example of a bar chart comparing the predicted and observed number of tuberculosis patients.

- Calibration can also be calculated using the Hosmer-Lemeshow test [85].

$$\text{Hosmer - Lemeshow test} = \frac{\Sigma\ (\text{observed no. of patients - predicted no. of patients})^2}{(\text{predicted number of patients})}$$

The calculated value of this test is compared with the value in the Chi-2 table for a (risk of 1ere species) = 0.05 and 18 ddl (degrees of freedom). The calibration is considered satisfactory given the absence of any significant difference between the predicted and observed risks. Using the example above, the Hosmer-Lemeshow test would be equal to $\frac{(1-2)2}{2} + \frac{(2-2)2}{2} + \frac{(2-3)2}{3} + \frac{(3-3)2}{3} + \ldots =$ = 1.28. We can conclude that the predicted number of TB patients and the observed number are not significantly different. The calibration of the predictive score for tuberculosis is therefore satisfactory.

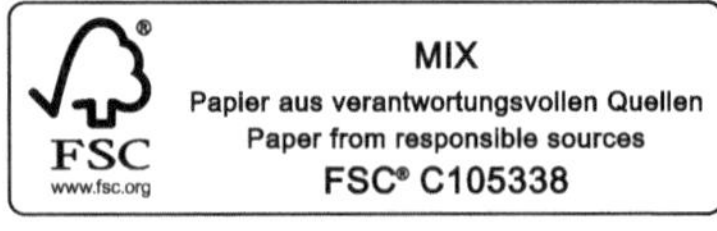

Printed by Books on Demand GmbH, Norderstedt / Germany